The Best Options
for
Diagnosing and Treating
Prostate Cancer

The Best Options
for
Diagnosing and Treating
Prostate Cancer

Based on research, clinical trials, and
scientific and investigational studies

by
James Lewis, Jr., Ph.D.
Survivor and Author

Health Education Literary Publisher
P.O. Box 948
Westbury, NY 11590
Telephone: (516) 942-5000
Email:JL3730@aol.com

Library of Congress Cataloging-in-Publication Data

Lewis, James, 1930–
     The best options for diagnosing and treating prostate
cancer : Based on research, clinical trials, and scientific and
investigational studies / by James Lewis, Jr.
         p.   cm.
     Includes bibliographical references and index.
     ISBN 1-883257-04-2
     1. Prostate—Cancer Popular works.   I. Title.
RC280.P7L485   1999   99.37185
616.99   463—dc21   CIP

Contents

FOREWORD

$\mathcal{J}$ust as I was beginning my training in Urology, I received a call from my father. I learned that "Uncle Jim" had been diagnosed with prostate cancer, and that he would like to call me to get some advice on the various treatment options. At this time, Dr. James Lewis was already an accomplished man. He had written many books and articles on the educational system, and he had always impressed me as being very bright and articulate. He also had an unwavering opinion regardless of how it was received by others. I was flattered that he would ask my advice, but also a little intimidated, and I knew that I had better know my stuff before I spoke with him.

When the call finally came, he presented all the relevant clinical facts and asked what I would recommend. Nearly eight years have past since that initial conversation, and with only minor modifications, the treatment I recommended for him then is still the treatment I would recommend for him now, given the same clinical information. Whether that reflects the effectiveness of the treatment I recommended, or the failure of the Urology and Radiation Oncology community to make any progress in the treatment of prostate cancer is open to debate.

Dr. Lewis presents what he believes to be "The Best Options for Diagnosing and Treating Prostate Cancer."

After reviewing the manuscript, it was clear that Dr. Lewis had done a very extensive review of the literature. While some of the conclusions are controversial, I feel that this book is a valuable source of information to the newly diagnosed man with prostate cancer. Moreover, his review of "The Best Complementary Therapy for Prostate Cancer Patients" is a must read for the practicing Urologist. The proliferation of non-traditional or complementary medical modalities is a reality that must be embraced by all physicians. Merely saying that herbal medication "may not help, but can't hurt," is not only inaccurate, but also may compromise patient care. In fact, the American Urological Association had a plenary session devoted to various nontraditional treatment options for BPH and Prostate Cancer.

"The Best Options for Diagnosing and Treating Prostate Cancer" is an example of Dr. Lewis' determination to help others with prostate cancer. It also reflects how the Internet makes information, that was once the near exclusive province of the physician, available to everyone. We as physicians should not feel threatened by these efforts; rather, we should welcome them. These efforts challenge us to keep up to date, and present us with a more informed patient who will still need our knowledge, clinical experiences, and expertise.

—Llewellyn M. Hyacinthe, M.D.

QUALIFYING STATEMENT

Neither the publisher nor the author of this book make or give the reader any warranty of the fitness of purpose for the information contained in this book. Nothing contained herein shall be deemed a specific recommendation of any particular drug or medical procedure, device, or method of medical treatment. You may not rely on any of the information contained herein for any purpose whatsoever other than for your general education. You must consult your own duly-licensed medical doctor for any medical problem you have. You must consult the pharmaceutical company that manufactures any particular drug or medication, in conjunction with your own medical doctor, as to the use or non-use of any particular drug or medication or medical treatment procedures. Statistical information contained in this book is also subject to several different interpretations. Do not rely upon any interpretation of statistical information contained in this book. You must have a qualified doctor assist you in the interpretation of this information.

In other words, although reasonable efforts have been made to ascertain the accuracy of statements made herein, neither the author nor the publisher make any promise or representation that any of the information in this publication is accurate or without errors or appropriate for any specific purpose or use. Readers should not rely upon any information contained herein where such reliance might cause loss or damage.

$\mathcal{I}$NTRODUCTION

$\mathcal{T}$ he purpose of my fourth book on prostate cancer is to make you aware of the best options for diagnosing and treating the disease. *The Best Options* is not intended to substitute for your physician. If your physician has another opinion, ask him or her to prove it by showing you the results of either a clinical trial or a scientific or investigational study. Your doctor should be able to substantiate his or her claims.

Be sure your doctor is staying abreast of new developments in the field of oncology and urology. As a prostate cancer adviser, I have witnessed too many doctors who have not kept up to date with what's happening in their profession. Don't permit these outdated doctors to jeopardize your life.

One physician I know of performed three biopsies on a patient without detecting any prostate cancer. Because the patient had an elevated PSA level, I subsequently advised him to undergo a 5-region biopsy. The patient went to his doctor, who said he had never heard of this technique. So I mailed the patient a clinical study, he shared it with the doctor, and the doctor subsequently conducted the 5-region biopsy and found the cancer. The patient was given a Gleason score of 8. Perhaps if the doctor had diagnosed the cancer at the time of the first biopsy, the patient might have received the proper treatment. Instead, by the time his cancer was finally diagnosed, he had developed a poorly differentiated tumor.

In another case, a patient told me has was going to undergo a radical prostatectomy. When he asked my opinion, I told him that I tended to be biased against surgery because I have heard of so many men whose cancer recurs after it. I advised him to undergo a spectroscopic MRSI to verify his doctor's opinion that he had stage T2C disease. But when the patient asked his doctor to give him a prescription for the diagnostic test, his doctor refused. The doctor felt that the MRSI was not necessary. Apparently, he was not knowledgeable about the test or its efficacy. Well, you can guess what happened. Several weeks after the operation, the patient received a pathologist's report indicating that he did not have stage T2C disease, but stage T3C. The cancer had spread to the his seminal vesicles. I reminded him that the MRSI would have shown seminal-vesicle involvement. If he had had this information, he would not have opted for surgery. To say the least, the patient is unhappy.

Very few physicians are willing to say that any one prostate cancer treatment is the "best." Instead, they will say it is "among the best" or "one of the best." I, on the other hand, am not reluctant to tell I am convinced something is the best, even when the so-called experts disagree with me. A "best choice" is defined as a procedure or treatment that offers a patient with prostate cancer the best chance of a cure. The choice may be supported by scientific evidence, a promising investigational study, or a survey. The choice may not be among those cited in the literature. It may not be the cheapest, and it may not be the most popular.

In some cases, physicians and scientists may disagree with the author. However, the author is not looking for popularity. Instead, he asks, does a treatment help patients? And, if so, what is the best way to use this treatment without harm to the patients. **My "best" selections are based primarily on the findings of various researchers and are presented in the ten chapters of this book.**

- Chapter 1 presents information on supplements that may prevent or delay a recurrence of prostate cancer.

- Most physicians and patients believe that the prostate-specific antigen (PSA) is the best marker for detecting prostate cancer. Chapter 2 makes the case that the ultra-sensitive PSA test is the best marker because it can detect prostate cancer one to 19 months before other clinical tests can—including the PSA test.

- Chapter 3 discusses an imaging test known as the magnetic resonance spectroscopic image (MRSI), which is designed to stage localized prostate cancer better than any other test. Patients should undergo the MRSI to pinpoint the exact location of localized disease prior to surgery.

- The sextant biopsy has been used by many physicians; however, one research group has now developed the 5-region biopsy, which uses the sextant process, but adds additional biopsies. As shown in Chapter 4, it has been found to detect 37 percent more cancer.

- Chapter 5 presents information on a form of radiation that is getting a great deal of attention from patients throughout the world: prostRcision. It is so named because its cure rate is reported to be similar to that of radical prostatectomy. When the side effects of prostRcision are compared with those of surgery, many find it preferable to the scalpel.

- At one time, when a patient's disease became hormonal-refractory, he usually had only a few years to live. However, today a complementary therapy—an herbal formula known as PC SPES—seems to be effective in prolonging the lives of 80 percent of patients. Chapter 1 presents details of this therapy.

- Not long ago, several studies reported that 80 percent of patients who underwent external beam radiation using photons had a recurrence of prostate cancer within 5 years. However, as chapter 7 shows, when combined with combination hormonal therapy, external beam radiation significantly increases survival time. As a result, all patients undergoing external beam radiation should seriously consider adding hormones to their treatment.

- As outlined in Chapter 8, the best method for detecting bone cancer is still the bone scan. However, the best treatment for finding bone cancer in multiple sites seems to be Quadramet.

- Prostate cancer patients treated with certain combinations of chemotherapy drugs had excellent results. Chapter 9 details these findings.

- Chapter 10 guides the patient in developing a sensible plan for diagnosing and treating his disease.

The chief reason for *The Best Options* is to make you a smarter patient so that you can engage in a meaningful discussion with your doctor to save or lengthen your life, to improve your quality of life, and to enable you to make effective diagnostic and treatment decisions. *The Best Options* is intended to be a powerful vehicle for you and your physician, one that will help you to understand and apply the choices together and join in a real partnership.

Remember, you are dealing with the most precious thing you have—your life. I know how hard it will be for you to make the best choice so that you come out as a winner against your bout with prostate cancer. None of us can afford to waste time, money, and energy being diagnosed with improper equipment or being treated with improper protocols.

I leave it up to you to examine my choices by researching opposing data in the library and on the Internet, so that you can arrive at the best choice. It's your body we are talking about, not mine or your doctor's. Use this book as a springboard to challenge any claims, and act according to your best judgment.

No doubt you will find some doctors who will discount a claim in order to mask their ignorance. For example, although the MRSI is covered in several medical texts, most physicians have never heard of it. Use this book to educate your doctors by sharing the research and findings with them.

Regardless of what you say, some doctors will discount the claims of this book just because I am not a medical doctor. However, I am a prostate cancer survivor, and I want the best for all my colleagues who are affected with this disease.

Because I advise thousands of prostate cancer patients each year, I am supposed to take an objective point of view in all matters related to the disease. However, sometimes it is difficult to do so. For example, I once made the claim to a urologist that the MRSI is the best technique for staging localized prostate cancer. He replied that I should not say that. I challenged him to give me one test, just one test, that has a positive predicted value of 97 percent. He had no defense.

On another occasion, I stated that PC SPES is the best therapy for hormone-refractory patients. Several physicians opposed me. I cried out, "Are you saying that chemotherapy can cure hormonal-refractory patients?" I got no response.

January, 1999
James Lewis, Jr., Ph.D.

Chapter 1

The Best Changes to Make to Possibly Prevent Prostate Cancer

Vitamins, Minerals, Supplements, Foods, Exercises, and Life Style Changes

Over the years, the medical community has given considerable attention to the cure of prostate cancer. However, for the most part, it has failed. Even this country's declaration of war on cancer has done little to wipe out this devastating disease. As a result, it appears that perhaps the most rational approach is not to try to cure prostate cancer, but rather to prevent it.

Throughout the world, a multitude of studies have shown that the lifestyle and environmental factors of each country are related to its incidence of prostate cancer. Recently, research on the chemical constituents of foods have indicated certain nutrients may be "protective" or "preventive" of prostate cancer. Additional studies have shown that vitamins, minerals, and other supplements play a role in prostate cancer.

The Basics of Prostate Cancer Chemoprevention

The development of prostate cancer is a process consisting of three steps:

1. A genetic alteration, called *initiation,* occurs in prostate cells.

2. This leads to the *promotion* of phenotypical changes in the cells and ultimately to the loss of replication, control, metastasis, and invasiveness.

3. This leads to *progression*, in which the prostate cells form malignant tumors with increased morphologic change.

The genetic alteration can be caused by hereditary or by damage from physical, viral, or chemical carcinogens. Promotion is usually caused by a physical or chemical influences. Some influences can act as initiator as well as promoter. In addition, other forces can encourage the progression of promoted cells.

Defining Chemoprevention

M.B. Sporn and his colleagues originally coined the term *chemoprevention* in 1976. They defined it as the use of natural or synthetic chemical agents to reverse, suppress, or prevent cellular progression to invasive cancer.

Cancer prevention is a theory and has yet to be proven. Well-designed clinical trials indicating a direct link between vitamins, minerals, and other supplements and the prevention of cancer still have to be completed.

Chemoprevention agents are immune enhancers that may be able to improve the body's ability to stop or delay the growth of prostate cancer. Immune enhancers function in at least four ways, some of which overlap:

1. They improve communication within the immune cells making them more efficient and powerful.

2. They increase the number of immune cells, making them more aggressive and more effective in fighting antigens.

3. They slow down and at times stop the production of free radicals.

4. In the long term, they significantly improve the environment within the blood and tissues where the immune cells work.

Although medicines are given to patients to make them well, some medicines actually depress the immune system. For example, a chemotherapeutic drug such as vinbilastine attempts to destroy or palliate prostate cancer cells, but it also depresses the immune system. Therefore, the long-term use of chemopreventive or chemo-suppressant supplements will strengthen the immune system and make the patient healthier.

Who Would Chemoprevention Benefit?

Chemoprevention inhibits or reverses prostate cancer by using noncytotoxic nutrients or pharmacologic compounds to protect the body from the development and progression of malignant cells.

Possible prostate cancer chemopreventive agents being investigated are diverse with regard to source, chemical structure, physiologic effects, vitamins, minerals, natural products, and synthetics. D.G. Bostwick identified the use of chemoprevention in prostate cancer as having a different end point of biomarker reduction rather than a pure reduction in prostate cancer incidence. Therefore, chemopreventive supplements would benefit the following patients:

1. Patients with high-grade prostatic intraepithelial neoplasia (PIN).

2. "Watchful waiting" patients.

3. Newly diagnosed patients awaiting definitive treatment.

4. Men at high risk of developing prostate cancer.

5. Men from the general population.

6. Posttreatment patients who wish to take chemoprevention supplements to prevent or delay the recurrence of prostate cancer

Chemopreventive Agents

The ideal chemopreventive agent should possess the following characteristics:

- It must be effective in preventing the development of prostate cancer.

- It must be free of both short- and long-term toxicity.

- It should be easily dispensed and ingested.

- It should be inexpensive.

The herbal formula PC SPES should be considered when evaluating a prostate cancer prevention program. The key to preventing prostate cancer involves enhancing the immune system as well as a supplement that will cause apoptosis.

Possible Chemoprevention Supplements

The same chemoprevention agents that seem to have an impact on the immune system also seem to prevent or destroy prostate cancer. Many of these supplements will be outlined in the following pages.

Vitamin A

Vitamin A is necessary for good health. Vitamin A is found in liver; various dairy products such as milk, cheese, butter, and ice cream; and in fatty fish such as herring, sardines, and tuna. It can also be found in the liver oils of shark, cod, and halibut. Vitamin A plays a part in cell differentiation, the process by which cells "mature." Differentiation helps prevent inappropriate growth, such as the controlled cell seen in cancer. Many studies in animals have shown that vitamin A and similar compounds decrease the incidence of cancer.

Vitamin C

Vitamin C plays a multifaceted role in the immune system. It is particularly abundant in white blood cells. These cells draw in foreign invaders such as bacteria and then destroy them using enzymes and free radicals. Vitamin C protects the cell itself from being damaged during this process. It also increases the production and function of other immune system components, including interferon (a biochemical messenger that promotes antiviral activity) and natural-killer cells (T cells that attack infected or cancerous cells).

Vitamin C acts as a powerful antioxidant, and it also enhances the immune system. It has been proven to have therapeutic benefits in a multitude of conditions—from macular degeneration, glaucoma, and cataracts to autoimmune diseases, infertility, and complications of pregnancy. Supplemental vitamin C speeds wound healing, protects the gums, slows the progression of arthritis, and reduces the complications of diabetes. It acts as an antihistamine, improves asthma and allergies, and in high intravenous doses is extremely effective in treating hepatitis and acute infections.

Prostate cancer begins when the DNA of a single cell is damaged or mutated and then replicates into a colony of abnormal, cancerous cells. A person's DNA takes thousands of damaging hits a day, yet only when the immune system is overwhelmed are the abnormal cells able to develop into full-blown cancer. Vitamin C both protects cellular DNA from free-radical damage and enhances the immune response that mops up these abnormal cells.

Numerous studies have demonstrated that high consumption of vitamin C-contained primarily in food, but also in supplements—is related to a decreased risk of cancer of the bladder, breast, cervix, colon, esophagus, mouth, lung, and pancreas. The research on vitamin C as a therapy for existing cancer is limited, yet provocative. In one study, Scottish physician Ewan Cameron, M.D., gave 10,000 mg of vitamin C daily to 294 cancer patients and observed 1,532 more who were not supplementing with vitamin C. The patients who took vitamin C survived almost twice as long as the control group.

Virtually all living organisms produce vitamin C. The exceptions are primates (including humans), guinea pigs, and Indian fruit-eating bats, all of whom must get this nutrient from their diets. Yet only one in 10 Americans eats the recommended five servings of fresh fruits and vegetables daily. Even five servings a day provide only 250 mg of the nutrient, and this doesn't take into account its fragility. When cooked or when cut and left sitting, fruits and vegetables lose about half their vitamin C content.

Vitamin D

When ingested in the body, vitamin D is converted into a related compound, alpha 25-D3, which is significantly more active than vitamin D. This form of vitamin D is available as a prescription medication called Calcitriol. Calcitriol has a multitude of benefits. When combined with calcium, it increases the ability of the stomach to absorb calcium and make oral calcium more effective. It will block the growth of prostate cancer when testosterone and dihydrotestosterone are present. When vitamin D is combined with vitamin A, these two vitamins seem to show considerable activity against prostate cancer cells. And vitamin D may be effective in both preventing and treating prostate cancer.

Vitamin E

It is not known why vitamin E might reduce the risk of prostate cancer. However, vitamin E is known to be an antioxidant, a compound that may prevent cancer from damaging DNA. In addition to its antioxidant activity, there are many other ways in which vitamin E works:

- It affects cell membranes.

- It may inhibit the proliferation of cells.

- It may stimulate the immune system or alter sex hormones.

- It may play a role in inhibiting or increasing apoptosis (cell death). In addition, it may play a role in differentiating and protecting the metabolic pathogens that rid the body of toxins.

A study conducted in Finland suggests that vitamin E can prevent prostate cancer. An analysis of this large prevention trial conducted by the National Cancer Institute (NCI) and the National Public Health Institute of Finland shows that long-term use of moderate doses vitamin E substantially reduced both the incidence of—and deaths from—prostate cancer in male smokers. The report was published in the March 18, 1998, issue of the *Journal of the National Cancer Institute* and the lead author is Olli P. Heinonen, M.D., D.Sc., of the Department of Public Health, University of Helsinki, Finland.

Known as the ATBC Study (Alpha-Tocopherol, Beta-Carotene Cancer Prevention Study, the trial showed that 50 to 69-year-old men who took 50 mg of alpha-tocopherol (a form of the antioxidant vitamin E) daily for 5 to 8 years had 32 percent fewer diagnoses of prostate cancer and 41 percent fewer prostate cancer deaths than did men who did not take vitamin E. The 50 mg dose of vitamin E is equal to about 50 IU and is about three times the Recommended Dietary Allowance. The 29,133 male smokers from Finland were randomly assigned to receive alpha-tocopherol, beta-carotene (20 mg), or a placebo daily.

Earlier results from the ATBC Study showed that men who took the beta-carotene supplement had 16 percent more cases of lung cancer and 14 percent more lung cancer deaths than did those who did not take beta-carotene. Men who drank large amounts of alcohol, and who took beta-carotene, had higher rates of lung cancer than did men who drank less alcohol. In the current analysis, men taking beta-carotene supplements had more prostate cancer as well, but this increase was not statistically significant and was limited to men who drank alcohol. Men taking both nutrients (beta-carotene and vitamin) had fewer cases of prostate cancer compared to men taking a placebo.

In men taking vitamin E, there was a reduction in clinically detectable prostate cancer beginning within two years of starting the supplement. This suggests that vitamin E may block a prostate tumor's progression. Most older men have microscopic areas of cancer in their prostate, few of which will progress to life-threatening disease.

Overall, men taking vitamin E had fewer diagnoses of later-stage cancers than did men not taking the supplement. The number of cancers diagnosed at earlier stages, when symptoms are few, was equivalent between supplement and placebo groups.

Beta-Carotene

Beta-carotene, which is found in plants, is a precursor of vitamin A. The body converts beta-carotene to vitamin A. Beta-carotene occurs mainly in fruits and vegetables that are deep yellow, orange, or dark green in color, such as carrots, squash, yams, peaches, apricots, spinach, collard or mustard greens, and broccoli. It is an antioxidant, a compound that may prevent cancer-causing substances from damaging DNA. Epidemiologic studies have linked a high intake of foods rich in beta-carotene and high serum levels of the micronutrient to a reduced risk of cancer. Beta-carotene stops the destruction of cells caused by oxidation; it also prevents the formation of free radicals. In one particular process, it relieves the stress on the immune system and slows down the aging process.

Selenium

Selenium is a nonmetallic trace element. A trace element is needed in minute amounts-in micrograms rather than milligrams. Selenium is essential in humans, but the body cannot manufacture it. Therefore, it must be supplied through the diet. The amount of selenium in food is directly related to the amount of selenium in the soil where the food is grown. Selenium levels vary greatly from region to region throughout the world; they can range from a total lack of selenium to a level that is so high, such as in some parts of China, that it is considered toxic. Some experts believe that year by year, selenium levels are declining which is disturbing considering the human body's need for selenium and the increase in cancer.

According to Larry C. Clark, Ph.D., of the University of Arizona School of Medicine in Tucson, more than 200 scientific studies involving humans have shown an association between relatively low selenium levels and an increased risk of developing cancer.

Selenium appears to combat cancer in three ways:

1. It acts in conjunction with glutathione peroxidase to protect cell membranes, and it expedites the repairing of damaged DNA molecules.

2. It inhibits the growth of tumors themselves.

3. It protects the liver, which is responsible for detoxifying the body, and it enables the liver to strengthen the immune system.

A 10-year trial conducted by Larry Clark et al. studied the effects of selenium supplementation on cancer prevention in patients with carcinoma of the skin. The study, which began in 1983, included a total of 1,312 skin cancer patients whose mean age was 63. They were seen at seven dermatology clinics in areas of the eastern United States where soil levels of selenium were relatively low. At that time, the primary purpose of the study was to determine whether dietary supplements of selenium could lower the incidence of basal-cell or squamous-cell skin cancers. In 1990, secondary purposes including the incidence of the most commonly occurring cancers-lung, prostate, and colorectal were added.

Patients in the double-blind randomized study (neither patients nor doctors knew who was receiving the selenium), took either a tablet containing 200 mcg of selenium as brewer's yeast, or a placebo, daily for 4.5 years. They were then followed for an additional 6.4 years. Three-quarters of the patients were men. The trial ended in January 1996.

The results showed that the total incidence of cancer was significantly lower in the selenium group than in the placebo group (77 cases versus 119), as was the incidence of some site specific cancers. The selenium group had fewer prostate cancers (13:35), a difference that is statistically significant. The results also showed that overall mortality was 17 percent less in the selenium group versus the control group (108:129), with this difference largely due to a 50 percent reduction in cancer deaths (29:57).

Tomatoes and Lycopene

Of all of the common carotenoids, lycopene is the most efficient scavenger of singlet oxygen. It is able to combat free radicals twice as efficiently as can beta-carotene. Current research suggests that lycopene's powerful antioxidant activity gives a high degree of protection against cholesterol oxidation, a process believed to influence prostate cancer. Epoxides, byproducts of the oxidation of cholesterol, measured in cancerous prostate tissue suggest that oxidized cholesterol is either a product of oxidative stress or that it has a direct carcinogenic effect. This antioxidant property may also protect both men and women from heart disease, as oxidation of LDL is one of the first steps in the development of atherosclerosis.

Researchers have also discovered that lycopene increases communication between cells. This mechanism, which allows healthy cells to communicate with each other, is lost during malignant transformation of cells. It is theorized that by restoring this communication process, lycopene may aid in reversing the malignant process.

Tomatoes, in addition to being a good source of a host of phytochemicals and antioxidants such as vitamins A and C, are also nature's richest source of lycopene, a red antioxidant carotenoid related to beta-carotene. Lycopene and beta-carotene are the predominant carotenoids in human tissue, and lycopene is the most abundant carotenoid found in prostate-gland tissue and serum. Lycopene, which is also found in watermelons, guavas, and pink grapefruits, is responsible for the red color associated with these fruits. The redder the color, the higher is the lycopene content, thus explaining why tomatoes are the richest source of this unique compound. One tomato has up to 10 mg of lycopene.

Although the protective effects of tomatoes were suggested earlier, a recently published study in the *Journal of the National Cancer Institute* found that men who consumed cooked tomato products were less likely to develop prostate cancer than were those who did not eat them. The study found that men who consumed 10 or more servings a week of tomato-based foods were up to 45 percent less likely to develop prostate cancer. Those men who ate four to seven portions per week reduced their chances for developing cancer by 20 percent.

In 1995, following the publication of a study by Edward Giovannucci, M.D., of the Harvard School of Public Health, identified a relationship between consumption of processed tomato products and a reduction in the risk of prostate cancer. These findings were expanded upon by Steven K. Clinton, M.D., Ph.D., of the Dana Farber Cancer Institute, who recently published clinical research supporting Dr. Giovannucci's evidence. "The data strongly suggests that tomato products should be a component of a healthy dietary pattern that includes at least five servings of fruits and vegetables per day," said Dr. Clinton. An additional study documenting the relationship between tomato consumption and a reduced risk of digestive tract and other cancers was presented by Carlo LaVecchia, M.D., of the Mario Negri Institute for Pharmacological Research in Milan. The health benefits of the Mediterranean diet are accounted for by extensive use of tomato products.

Modified Citrus Pectin

A compound derived from citrus fruits, modified citrus pectin, may provide a means of reducing or preventing the spread of prostate cancer. Pectin is a branched-chain carbohydrate found in plant cell walls, that hold adjacent cells together. All plants contain pectin, and apples and citrus fruits are particularly rich in it. Modified citrus pectin (MCP) is made from breaking the large pectin molecules into shorter and less-branched chains and partially degrading the carbohydrates.

Special proteins called *lectins* occur on cell surfaces and are used for communication with other cells. Cells interact when their lectins combine with structurally complementary forms on other cells. There are many kinds of lectins. One particular family of lectins has an affinity for galactose, and hence are called *galectins*. Certain cancer cells are especially rich in galectins and interact with other cells by bonding to galactose. By this means, a cancer cell that detaches from a primary tumor and enters the blood or lymph system can attach to a vascular endothelial cell far away from the primary site and begin a new tumor. This is the process of *metastasis*. MCP has particularly high amounts of the sugar galactose, which may be responsible for its ability to greatly reduce metastasis in animals.

An encouraging study published in the *Journal of the National Cancer Institute* showed that treating melanoma cells with MCP prevented them from forming new tumors. Melanoma cells were grown in culture and incubated with either no additions or with MCP. The melanoma cells were injected into the tail veins of mice. After 17 days, the mice were autopsied, and the tumors in their lungs (the site of metastasis) were counted. The group receiving cells incubated with no additions averaged 33 lung tumor colonies per mouse. But mice receiving MCP-treated melanoma cells had no lung tumors. This suggested that MCP had covered up the melanoma cells' binding sites, making them unable to attach to other cells.

Oral consumption of MCP may reduce metastasis in rats injected with prostate cancer cells, and it may have the same effect on the metastasis of human cancers. Some studies suggest that human cancer-cell lines—including prostate cancer cells treated with MCP may have greatly reduced adhesion to an endothelial base in vitro. It bounds sites on the cancer cells that otherwise might have attached to blood vessel cells.

Pecta-Sol modified citrus pectin was given to 35 patients with different kinds of cancer at the Pine Street Clinic. The patients were then tracked over the course of a year and a half to determine, first, if they currently had metastatic sites away from the primary site of their cancer, and second, if new sites appeared local to the primary site or distant to the site. During the study, the patients continued their conventional cancer treatment. Dosage was 15 gm per day administered orally. The presence of metastasis was determined by independent conventional medical assessment (e.g., MRI, palpitation), and the timing of metastatic examination was also independently prescribed.

In another study, 18 men (ages 48–77) with diagnosed prostate cancer consumed 15 gm of Pecta-Sol per day for 18 months. Nine men had metastasis outside the prostate at the beginning of the trial. Of these nine, two continued to develop new metastatic sites throughout an 18-month period. One other person developed new sites after 7 months of MCP consumption. Subject to the limitations of recording, 15 men showed no sign of new metastatic development between month 7 and month 18.

Of nine men without metastasis at the beginning of the study, six had no metastases during the 18-month period; two had new localized metastasis at one point during the first seven months; and one had distant and local metastasis during the first seven months. None developed metastases after 7 months of consuming MCP.

Soy Products

In China, the word for soybean is *ta-tou*, which means "greater bean." This is not surprising given the importance soybeans play in Asian culture, both as a food and as a medicine. In the West, for the past several decades, the soybean has been the focus of research into its institutional and medical benefits. There is sufficient scientific data to suggest that the much lower mortality rates in Asian countries from a number of degenerative diseases, such as prostate cancer and breast cancer, correlate with high consumption of soy. The human body makes very good use of the bean's nutrients (proteins, vitamins, minerals) as well as the phytochemicals such as isoflavones, saponins, protease inhibitors, and phytosterols. Science has thoroughly established the beneficial role of these phytochemicals.

There are two major issues to be concerned with when planning soy use. First, establish the quality of soybeans selected, as well as the care with which blending, milling, and extracting are performed. High concentrations of isoflavones and genisteins for the nourishment and strengthening of the immune system can only be achieved with quality raw materials and careful manufacture. Secondly, how do we provide the body with enough valuable soy nutrients if it hasn't the capacity to absorb them? When the immune system is negatively affected by a degenerative disease like prostate cancer or breast cancer, the digestive system is compromised. And where medical treatment has affected the intestinal tract (which often happens with radiation and chemotherapy), a problem of body absorption arises.

The impact of soybean on PSA levels was tested for 150 days in a clinic that uses an integrative medical approach to treat prostate cancer. Patients were not on radiation, chemotherapy, or hormonal treatment during the recording period, and they followed a customized nutritional protocol. At a daily dosage of one 250-ml bottle of fermented soy drink per day (reduced later in the protocol), encouraging results were found:

Ecogen 851™ Tracking Statistics

#	Patient Initials	Age	PSA	Start	60	90	120	150	% Drop	Stage	Cell
				PSA Value After x Days							
1	ES	56	34	29	27	21	17*	17	50.0%	B1	Tetrap
2	WT	59	42	31	28	19	13	20	52.4%	C	Aneu
3	PP	66	12	11	7	5	5*	5	58.3%	B1	Tetrap
4	TH	62	8	5	5	5	4*	5	37.5%	A3	Dipl
5	MB	77	7	7	6.5	6	6*	6	14.3%	A1	Dipl
6	JG	65	28	27	22	15	11	10*	64.3%	B1	Tetrap
7	HS	59	16	10	10	8	6.5*	7	56.3%	A3	Tetrap
8	KM	39	39	32	32	24	19	15*	61.5%	C	Aneu
9	DM	66	12	14	14	12			0.0%	C	Aneu
10	MG	54	6	5	5	4			33.3%	B1	Tetrap
11	GF	49	7	7	8	7	7*		0.0%	A1	Dipl
12	LC	53	16	13	12	8*			50.0%	A3	Tetrap
13	BL	55	8	9	9	9			-12.5%	B1	Tetrap
14	LS	61	22	24	21	20	20	16	27.3%	B2	Dipl
Average					18.36	11.64	10.85	11.22			
Drop from Initial PSA Average					-37%	-41%	-39%				

* indicates reduction to half-bottle per day

Among the 14 individuals in the study, PSA levels had dropped 37 percent at the end of 90 days. Ten men studied for 120 days had a 41 percent decline in PSA, and nine men followed for 150 days had an average drop of 39 percent.

Therefore, fermented soy is recommended for those whose digestion is compromised by disease, aggressive therapy, or surgery. It provides a proven way to increase nutrition and a dependable source of bioavailable "free" aglycone soy isoflavones. Soybean isoflavone-concentrate products offer preventive support and maintenance of the immune system. The two can be taken together to help repair and strengthen an immune system.

Green Tea

Green tea is produced when black tea leaves are steamed and dried. Because the leaves aren't permitted to ferment and oxidize, many of their nutrients are preserved, particularly the polyphenols. The strong, astringent flavor of green tea is due to its polyphenol content. Polyphenols, antioxidants that seem to increase the activity of antioxidant enzymes, seem to be more potent than vitamin C and E.

Approximately 30 percent of a green tea leaf is composed of polyphenols.

Polyphenols combat cancer in three ways: (1) they can stop the formation of cancer cells, (2) they turn up the body's natural detoxification defenses, and (3) they suppress cancer advancement. Green tea seems to attack specific cancer types in a preventive and therapeutic mode.

The four primary polyphenols in green tea are: (1) epicatechin (EC), (2) epicatechin gallate (ECG), (3) epigallocatechin (EGC), (4) and epigallocatechin gallate (EGCG). These chemicals, in green tea especially EGCG, have been carefully studied by scientists and found to be responsible for anticancer activity. Shutsung Liao, Ph.D., and several other investigators created experimental human prostate tumors in laboratory mice. They then treated the mice with EGCG, ECG, or one of the other two polyphenols. They found that 1 mg of EGCG injected daily into the body cavity prevented initial tumors from progressing and shrunk some existing tumors by 60 to 70 percent within two weeks. The amazing results demonstrated that EGCG had a powerful antitumor effect.

Coenzyme Q-10

Enzymes are protein molecules responsible for the body's metabolic functions. They join up molecules, causing some to be created and some to be degraded. They also make it possible to speed up thousands of chemical reactions taking place simultaneously with the cells. A molecule cannot react unless it connects with another molecule; an enzyme is a necessary biological catalyst. Although an enzyme joins two types of molecules over and over, it is not involved with any other process at this stage.

Every enzyme is coupled to one or two coenzymes, smaller molecules without which most enzymes cannot function. Therefore, most molecules that are being built by an enzyme cannot be completed unless the necessary coenzyme is present. Vitamins are often the coenzymes of various enzymes. The body's cell system will begin to fail if a particular coenzyme is absent. Coenzyme Q-10 (Co-Q-10) is vital to the production of energy in the human body. Co-Q-10 is also an essential compound of the mitochondrial membranes. Mitochondria are intracellular structures that produce adenosine triphosphate, the basic energy molecule. They extract about 95 percent of the total energy from food, use the food molecules, stored chemical energy to pump protons across the mitochondrial membrane, and produce energy from carbohydrates and lipids in almost all cells in the body. Because coenzyme Q-10 plays a critical role, sufficient amounts must be available to sustain life.

A scientific study by the late Karl Folkers, M.D., indicated that coenzyme Q-10 may have positive effects on prostate cancer. The study involved 15 men all of whom failed conventional treatment and had a rising PSA. They were given 200 mg of coenzyme Q-10 three times a day. One patient who had metastatic cancer died. Ten of the remaining patients experienced shrinking of their prostate gland, and achieved a stabilized PSA level within 100 days.

D. W. V. Judy, M.D., one of the investigators, said patients should avoid the dry supplement and instead use the oil-based formulation because it remains in the body longer. Co-Q-10 does, however, improve the immune response of the existing cells.

It appears that Co-Q-10 provides multiple benefits. It is an effective agent against heart disease, high blood pressure, and periodontal disease; it slows aging; and it may be an agent against prostate cancer.

Garlic

Garlic has been shown to protect lipids (fats and cholesterol in the blood) from being oxidized, thus, preventing the beginning of free-radical formation, which causes many cancers. In fact, garlic extracts have been shown to decrease the development of cancer even after exposure to radiation and other carcinogens. It is believed garlic (1) plays a role in detoxifying carcinogens; (2) enhances the liver's ability to metabolize and neutralize carcinogens that would produce cancer cells and tumors; and (3) stimulates the liver to more effectively identify carcinogens and convert them into water-soluble compounds. Garlic may also block the effects of certain groups of fatty acids called mostaglandins, which may encourage tumors to develop when they are left unchecked. A compound derived from aged garlic (garlic stores commercially for at least a year) may dramatically diminish the growth of prostate cancer cells.

Researchers at Memorial Sloan-Kettering Cancer Center in New York studied cells that retained many of the features of the diseased prostate. For instance, they multiplied faster when exposed to testosterone, the primary male sex hormone, or to DHT, a far more potent analog produced from testosterone.

The cultured cells also produced compounds characteristic of human prostate tumors, making them a good model of human disease. The researchers exposed the cells to S-allylmercaptocysteine (SAMC), a sulfur compound that forms as garlic ages. The SAMC caused the cancer cells to break down testosterone two to four times more quickly than normal—and through a route that does not produce DHT. In essence, the garlic derived compound did the same thing that testosterone deprivation would do.

At concentrations that could develop in the blood of people taking commercially marketed aged-garlic pills, the SAMC slowed the cancer cells' growth as much as 70 percent, when compared to untreated cells.

SAMC cut the production of two proteins exuded by the cells (including PSA) and often used in blood tests for prostate cancer. The garlic-induced PSA decrease was greater than expected, out of proportion to the decrease in cancer growth, which might further retard a tumor growth.

Shitake Mushroom

Shitake mushroom is a wide flat-capped mushroom. Although grown primarily in Asia, it is used throughout the United States and Europe. It is high in protein (13–18 percent) and contains compounds such as niacin, thiamine, riboflavin, and a polysaccharide called *Lentinar*. Lentinar is approved in Japan as an anticancer drug. Recent research has shown that Lentinar stimulates macrophages and natural-killer cells to destroy cancer cells and tumors. Another substance isolated in shitake mushrooms, *cortinelin*, has been found to be an effective broad-spectrum antibiotic. Studies in the United States and Japan have shown that the shitake mushroom is a cancer fighter as well as a booster of the immune system.

Reishi Mushroom

A mushroom used traditionally in China reishi mushroom is similar to the shitake mushroom as it enhances the immune system. It causes lymphocytes to multiply rapidly when encountering disease-causing agents and to trigger production of interleukin-2. Reishi mushroom also acts to promote the creation of adhesion molecules that help to collect immune cells in a specific location in the body where they may be needed. Reishi mushroom also stimulates antitumor activity.

MGN-3

Dr. Mamdott Ghoneum perfected MGN-3 with the Department of Immunology at Drew University in Los Angeles, California. MGN-3 is produced by integrating, through hydrolysis, extracts from the outer shell of rice bran with the extracts from three different mushrooms: shitake (yielding lentinan), kawartake (yielding krestin), and soehirotkae (yielding sizo firan). By itself, rice bran exhibits fairly strong antiviral effects. Extracts from these three mushrooms have been shown to have anticancer properties.

The immune system is comprised of more than 130 subsets of white blood cells. Natural-killer (NK) cells are composed of about 15 percent white blood cells. They provide the first line of defense for combating any invading body. Each white blood cell contains several small granules, which function as "ammunition." When an NK cell recognizes a cancer cell, it attaches itself to the outer membrane of the cell, injecting granules directly in the body of the cell. The granules then "explode," causing destruction of the cancer cells. The process is repeated over and over. If the immune system is healthy, NK cells may take on two cancer cells.

MGN-3's primary function is to enhance the activity of the immune system so that it is capable of doing its job.

There appear to be five ways in which MGN-3 improves the immune system:

1. It increases the number of explosive granules in NK cells. The more granules there are, the more cancer cells it can destroy.

2. It increases interference levels by inhibiting the replication of viruses and other parasites, and it increases NK-cell activity.

3. It increases the formation of tumor necrosis factor, a protein that helps to fight cancer cells.

4. It increases NK activity by 300 percent (or more).

5. The oral ingestion of MGN-3 increases the activity of key immune cells, like T cells, by 200 percent and B cells by 250 percent.

MGN-3 works fast and without any toxicity. After 16 hours, NK-cell activity increased 1.3 to 1.5 times. After one week, NK activity increased eightfold. NK activity continued to increase, and after the end of two months, NK-cells were killing 27 times more cancer cells in a 4-hour period than they were prior to ingesting MGN-3.

A study conducted by Dr. Ghoneum involved 27 cancer patients, ranging in age from 42 to 59, who had several different types of cancer, including breast, cervical, prostate, leukemia, and multiple myeloma. All patients had low NK-cell activity at the beginning of the study. After only two weeks, the NK activity had increased 174 to 385 percent. In another study involving three prostate cancer patients, two of the three had complete remission and a decline in their PSA levels. One reached a normal level after a month: another was normal after 2 months: and the third patient's PSA level dropped from 87.2 to 7 ng/ml after 4 months.

Foods That Might Help Prevent Prostate Cancer

Cruciferous Vegetables

Broccoli, cabbage, kale, brussel sprouts, collard, mustard greens, and watercress are called cruciferous vegetables. They contain compounds called *phytochemicals* and *indoles* that may prevent cancer. Cruciferous vegetables are rich sources of another cancer fighter, *sulforaphane*, a potent trigger for detoxifying tissues and blood, and for promoting cancer-preventive enzymes.

Cruciferous vegetables, especially watercress, contain *phenethyl isothiocyrnate*, which has been shown to inhibit certain tumors in animals.

Fruits

Citrus fruits contain compounds called *limonoids,* which stimulate the production of certain types of enzymes. Most fruits contain bioflavonoids and antioxidants.

Recommended Supplemental Dosage

Modified citrus pectin	2 tsp (13 gm) in water daily
Green tea	Four or more cups daily
Coenzyme Q-10	200 mg three times daily
Vitamin D	400 IU daily
Garlic, raw or cooked	Three or more times per week
Shitake mushroom	Two to six servings per week

MGN-3	12 capsules (250 mg) per day for two weeks, then 4 capsules per day
Vitamin E	400 mg twice a day
Selenium	400 mcg twice daily* *Important: Selenium can be toxic at extremely high dosages. If you are taking selenium and experience hair or fingernail loss, see your physician immediately.
Tomato and lycopene	No recommend dosage
Soybeans & soybean products	At least 35 gm per day
Reishi mushroom	Two to four servings per week
Soy phytochemicals	At least 50 gm per day
Cruciferous vegetables	At least one serving of these vegetables daily
Fruits, various	At least five daily servings
Vitamin C	125 mg twice a day
Vitamin A	500 IU three times a day

More Evidence

The *Journal of the National Cancer Institute* (Vol. 901, No. 21, November 4, 1998) reported on a study of nutrition and socioeconomic factors in relation to prostate cancer deaths. It reached the following conclusions:

- The intake of cereals, soybeans, and nuts and/or seeds, and fish are negatively associated with prostate cancer mortality.

- Prostate cancer mortality is positively associated with diet.

- Intake of energy, total fat, and animal products (milk, meat, and poultry) were positively associated with prostate cancer mortality.

- Unlike meat and poultry, fish appears to protect against prostate cancer.

- The omega-3 fatty acids appear to inhibit the growth of prostate cancer tumors.

- A strong correlation exists between energy from fish and soy products.

- Energy from soybeans is inversely associated with prostate cancer mortality.

- On a per-unit energy basis (kilocalories), soy effect was the largest in the dataset.

- Eating tofu is associated with a decreased risk of prostate cancer.

- Vegetables and the consumption of cereals are associated with a reduced risk of cancer.

- Consumption of cereal is inversely related to prostate cancer.

- The combined effect of both insottavonods and lignins, per their dieting sources of soy, legumes, cereal, and vegetables, may protect against prostate cancer.

- Consumption of whole milk is strongly and positively associated with prostate cancer mortality.

- The protection afforded by cereal intake is more strongly related to prostate cancer mortality than is the intake of meat and milk.

Don't Fight Prostate Cancer With Supplements Alone

To support the immune system, dietary supplements should not be used by themselves. Other immunity boosters must also be employed as discussed below:

1. Exercise moderately at least 30 minutes a day for four to seven days a week.

2. Establish a positive attitude and support by establishing a genuinely supportive relationship with others.

3. Join a support group.

4. Keep a diary.

5. Eat a healthy diet and include the supplements described in this chapter.

6. Maintain balance in life. Avoid undermining the immune system with negative energy.

7. Reduce stress by prayer, meditation, relaxing, trying biofeedback, laughing more, taking a warm bath, breathing deeply, getting a massage, and undergoing accupressure.

Why These Supplements and Foods Were Chosen

The supplements in this chapter were chosen because:

1. They were supported by multiple studies and in a multiple-national study.

2. Some of the studies were performed with rats and/or human beings.

3. Most of the supplements are known to enhance the immune system.

4. Not only did the cross-national study include diet: it also included prostate cancer mortality rates, a composite of other health-related factors, sanitation, and economic variables.

5. The multiple-national study was generally consistent with previous studies.

6. Multiple-national data also included the United States.

How You May Use This Information

Follow the recommendations below:

1. Eat a diet *low* in fat.
   - Eat fish instead of red meat and chicken.

   - Eat fresh vegetables, whole grains, soybeans, and whole grain snacks.

2. Take the recommended vitamins, minerals, and other supplements.

3. Eat herbs and condiments, especially the following:
   - Cooked or raw garlic three to four times weekly.

   - At least one to eight cups of green tea daily.

   - One serving of cruciferous vegetables daily.

   - Two to three shitake or reishi mushrooms two or three times a week.

   - Soybeans, tofu, tempeh, and other soy products four to six times a week.

4. Practice balance.

- Don't overeat.

- Avoid overexercising.

5. Eat three to four vegetables daily, including root vegetables, leafy green vegetables, carrots, squash, brussels sprouts, broccoli, and collard greens.

Chapter 2

THE BEST TUMOR MARKER FOR MONITORING PROSTATE CANCER AFTER TREATMENT

Ultrasensitive PSA

The best tumor marker for monitoring prostate cancer patients for a recurrence after treatment should meet several essential criteria:

1. There should be evidence of treatment failure after the initial therapy.

2. There should be a possible recurrence of the disease.

3. Immediate pretreatment should be warranted.

4. The test should be inexpensive.

5. The test should reveal the recurrence sooner than a clinical study.

If all of these criteria are fulfilled, monitoring for a recurrence should result in both the early discovery of treatment failure and a decrease in morbidity and mortality from the disease process. The current serum PSA test, because of its limited detection rate, fails to meet all of these criteria. To detect early recurrence of prostate cancer, a PSA test must be perfected that will signal treatment failure much earlier than will the standard PSA test.

Prostatic Specific Antigen (PSA)

Physicians and researchers in this country and abroad have accepted the prostate-specific antigen (PSA) as the best marker for detecting and treating prostate cancer.

In 1986, the Food and Drug Administration (FDA) approved the PSA blood test (1) as a diagnostic tool for determining whether treatment for prostate cancer had eliminated the disease and (2) as a technique for monitoring a patient for a recurrence. In 1994, the FDA approved using the PSA test to detect prostate cancer. In addition, researchers and physicians have used PSA levels for: estimating the time to clinical failure after treatment; calculating the rate of change in a patient's cancer cell; helping to estimate a patient's pathological stage and to determine if there is lymph-node involvement; monitoring any recurrence of prostate cancer; and separating patients with benign prostatic hyperplasia (BPH) from those with prostate cancer.

Ultrasensitive PSA Assay

The ultrasensitive PSA assay allow for the detection of much lower concentrations of PSA than does the standard PSA assays. The (FDA) has approved the IMX-PSA assay of

Abbott Laboratories, and it is commercially available. The IMX-PSA correlates well with the Tandem-R assay manufactured by Hybritech. The minimal detectable level of the IMX-PSA assay is 0.03 ng/ml. A third Hybritech assay may have an even lower detection level, 0.004 ng/ml. In eight patients who underwent radical prostatectomy and later experienced a recurrence (using 0.1 ng/ml to indicate treatment failure) the PSA level provided from several months to 3 years of lead time. The ability to detect tumor recurrence after surgery using an ultrasensitive PSA allows for early institution of adjuvant therapy.

Nichols Institute Ultrasensitive PSA

The Nichols Institute has introduced an ultrasensitive PSA with a sensitivity level of 0.007 ng/ml, but it only reports 0.02 ng/ml compared to 0.01 ng/ml for other sensitive assays. This enables Nichols to detect a recurrence of prostate cancer much sooner than other tests can. After radical prostatectomy patients with measurable PSA levels (0.1 ng/ml) have been shown to have a recurrence within 20 months. The average time for the ultrasensitive PSA to increase was 0.02 ng/ml per month. Therefore, several measurements of PSA using an ultrasensitive PSA have been known to detect a recurrence of prostate cancer after surgery several months earlier than the standard test. If early determination of a recurrence of prostate cancer can be made, then re-treatment can begin.

The Journal of Urology, (Vol. 149, 787–792, April 1993) reported the results of a study titled "Early Detection of Residual Prostate Cancer after Radical Prostatectomy by an Ultrasensitive Assay for Prostatic Specific Antigen" conducted at the Department of Urology at Stamford University School of Medicine. Thomas A. Stamey, M.D., and colleagues evaluated the usefulness of an ultrasensitive PSA modified from the standard Young Pros-Check PSA test with a biological detecting limit at 0.07 ng/ml. The purpose of this test was to detect residual prostate cancer at an earlier date. The researchers studied retrospectively a number of frozen serum samples taken after radical prostatectomy from 22 patients who had residual prostate cancer with detectable PSA levels of 0.3 ng/ml or greater as measured by the standard PSA test. The central groups consisted of 33 cystoprostatectomy patients who had bladder cancer, but not prostate cancer, and 23 patients who had a higher probability for a cure. All controlled patients (282 of 283 samples or 96%) without prostate cancer had PSA value of less than 0.1 ng/ml.

The ultrasensitive value of 0.1 ng/ml is considered the residual prostate cancer limit. In the 22 patients with a recurrence of prostate cancer, the ultrasensitive PSA test detected the recurrence with a PSA of 0.1 ng/ml or greater much earlier than did the standard PSA test (0.3 ng/ml or greater). On screening 187 post-radical prostatectomy patients without evidence of prostate cancer, (i.e., PSA level of 0.1 ng/ml or less) the results of the study indicated that the ultrasensitive PSA test detects residual or recurrent prostate cancer after surgery much earlier than does the standard PSA test. As a result, early detection of residual prostate cancer may improve long-term survival for patients by allowing them to undergo adjuvant therapy.

Understanding the Advantages of the Ultrasensitive PSA Test

There are several advantages to undergoing the ultrasensitive PSA test instead of the standard PSA test. These include:

1. A recurrence of prostate cancer can be detected earlier.

2. It can be used by a physician to determine the doubling time of the PSA, thus giving the doctor

sufficient time to decide when and how to re-treat the patient.

3. It can be used to diagnose prostate cancer.

4. It can be used to help assess the stage of a tumor.

5. Some ultrasensitivity tests can detect a recurrence of prostate cancer six months to ten months before the standard PSA assay.

How You May Use This Information

1. Instead of having the standard PSA test, consider having the ultrasensitive PSA test in order to monitor your response after treatment.

2. Decide on an ultrasensitive PSA sensitivity limit for use in other treatment areas, such as external beam radiation, cryosurgery, and brachyherapy.

Chapter 3

THE BEST CHOICE FOR STAGING LOCALIZED PROSTATE CANCER

Combined MRI and Spectroscopic MRI (MRSI)

Before the clinical use of the prostate-specific antigen (PSA) test became widespread, most organ-confined prostate cancer was discovered by a digital rectal exam (DRE) or during a transurethral resection (TRUP). While use of the PSA test increased the detection rate of prostate cancer, revealing cancer that would not have been detected by a DRE, there was no effective way to pinpoint its exact location. Although imaging studies to determine tumor size and location would be invaluable in the clinical staging of the disease, most methods (except for the combined MRI and MRSI) were not sufficient to be useful for most patients. The positive and negative predictive values for the detection of extracapsular extension and seminal vesical invasion with either computed tomography, endorectal ultrasound, or body coil MRI are believed to be too low to base treatment decisions on. Doctors typically reviewed the PSA, Gleason score, and other conditions of the patient and then made an educated guess about his stage. As a result, doctors were incorrect 50 to 60 percent of the time, causing the patient a great deal of anxiety-and money. To improve their "batting average", physicians began referring to the Partin Tables, which cite at an 85 percent probability the location or how extensive the disease is.

The Importance of Staging

A patient's prostate cancer must be staged before any decision can be made regarding his treatment. Staging is based on the extent of the primary tumor, the pathologic examination of the tissue, whether cancer is found in the lymph nodes,/and whether the patient has metastatic disease.

Clinical staging is done preoperatively using laboratory tests, including biopsy, and a physical examination of the patient. *Pathologic staging* is done by assessing surgically removed tissues and organs; it often exceeds the clinical estimation of the extent of the disease.

The Goal of Treating Localized Prostate Cancer

The goal of treating clinically localized prostate cancer is to cure it: that is, as stated at a recent prostate cancer meeting in Antwerp, Belgium, to give the patient the best chance of dying of something else. A number of factors should be considered when deciding whether a patient is suitable for such therapy. Chief among them is pinpointing the location of the cancer. While it may be impossible to determine the location with a 100 percent accuracy, physicians should certainly attempt to do so.

The Illumination Areas of Combined MRI/MRSI

Tumor volume refers to the size of the tumor and is often indicated in centimeters. *Organ-confined* refers to cancer that is located within the prostate gland or capsule. This location has the best cure rate. *Capsular penetration* refers to the spread of the tumor beyond the prostate gland. The extent of penetration is defined in terms of maximum length of the tumor that has penetrated the capsule. If the cancer has affected the seminal vesicles, there is often cancer at other sites in the body. The combination of (1) the high-specificity of MRSI to metabolically identify prostate cancer with (2) the high sensitivity of pelvic phased-array/endorectal-coil MRI has allowed for the improved assessment of the location and extent of cancer within the prostate and the possibility of spread of cancer outside the gland.

Components of the Spectroscopic MRI

Modified MRI

Magnetic resonance imaging (MRI) uses a magnetic field and radio-frequency waves to noninvasively obtain anatomic pictures (images) forced on tissue water. The images can be contrasted so that the cancer appears as a reunion of low signal intensity when compared to surrounding regions of healthy tissue. The degree of signal intensity is due to changes in the structure of the normal tissue. In the case of prostate cancer, prostatic ducts (sacs containing prostatic fluids) are replaced with densely packed, cancerous epithelial cells. However, in some cases, the diagnosis of cancer based on an MRI is erroneous because factors other than cancer can cause a decrease in signal intensity (e.g., postbiopsy hemorrhage, chronic prostatitis, benign prostatic hyperplasia, intraglandular dysplasia, trauma, and therapy). These factors can limit definitive diagnosis by MRI alone, and in some cases, they can lead to overestimation of tumor presence and capsular penetration.

The endorectal coil combined with the four external coils is used to acquire anatomic images with much higher resolution than what was previously possible. The endorectal coil provides the necessary sensitivity to focus on the prostate and surrounding structures. The pelvic phased-array (for external coil 5) allows for a larger field of view in order to assess the pelvic lymph nodes and bones for metastatic disease. Improving the magnetic resonance technology has allowed for a reduction in the time required for this component.

The endorectal/pelvic phased-coil MRI alone is quite accurate in detecting seminal-vesicle invasion and the spread of prostate cancer outside the capsule (96% and 81%, respectively). However, localization of cancer cells within the prostate by MRI alone is limited because factors such as chronic prostatitis, benign prostatic hyperplasia, interglandular dysplasia, trauma and therapy can cause a decrease in signal intensity.

MR Spectroscopic Imaging

The development of MR spectroscopic imaging (MRSI) has expanded the diagnostic assessment beyond the anatomic information provided by the MRI. The MRSI uses a magnetic field and radiowaves to noninvasively obtain metabolic pictures (spectra) based on the relative concentrations of cellular chemicals (metabolites). The MRSI provides metabolic information specific to the prostate through detection of the cellular metabolites citrate, creatine, and choline.

Using the same endorectal/pelvic phased coil technology for imaging, three-dimensional phased-encoded spectroscopic studies have become possible. The entire prostate can be evaluated in one study, and excellent images can be obtained from volumes as small as 0.24 ml. As a result, by superimposing the spectroscopic three-dimensional dataset on corresponding images, the exact location of the tumor may be determined and the volume estimated.

The endorectal/pelvic phased-coil MRI alone is quite accurate in detecting seminal-vesicle invasion and the spread of prostate cancer outside the capsule (96% and 81%, respectively). However, localization of cancer within the prostate by MRI alone is limited because factors such as chronic prostatitis, benign prostatic hyperplasia, intra-glandular dysplasia, trauma and therapy can cause a decrease in signal intensity.

Some Advantages of combined MRI/MRSI

The addition or MRSI to MRI has already demonstrated several advantages to the use of MRI as outlined in the following:

- MRSI will probably have the greatest impact on the assessment of prostate cancer therapy and on the selection of additional therapy, since therapy often causes structural changes that limit assesment of other modalities such as MRI and ultrasound which rely on structural changes to identify cancer.

- Scientists have already shown that the MRSI can distinguish residual or recurrent prostate cancer from normal and necrotic tissue after cryosurgery. They also have evidence that the same is true for other therapies such as hormone ablation, radiation, and chemotherapy and that the MRSI can detect residual cancer in the prostatic bed after radical prostatectomy.

- MRSI data are useful in guiding biopsies in patients with consistently rising PSA levels but negative biopsies. The MRSI covers the entire gland, whereas biopsies sample only a small fraction of the gland, often missing neoplasms.

- Postbiopsy hemorrhage, a major impediment to MRI interpretation, occurs frequently in prostate cancer patients. It occurred in 28 percent of all patients studied and was extensive (involving more that 50% of the sites sampled in 63% of these patients).

- The addition of an MRSI sequence to an MRI staging exam significantly increased specificity and accuracy of tumor detection in the presence of postbiopsy hemorrhage.

- A review of MR data has suggested that the addition of MRSI can improve staging of prostate cancer prior to therapy. Studies on MRI/MRSI staging after therapy are ongoing.

- In a preliminary study of 85 prostate cancer patients who have a combined MRI/MRSI exam prior to radical prostatectomy, significantly higher choline levels and significantly lower citrate levels were observed in regions of cancer as compared to BPH and normal prostatic tissues. The ratio of these metabolites (choline/citrate) in regions of cancer had minimal overlap with normal and BPH values.

- In a preliminary study of 25 patients before and after cryosurgery, MRSI was able to distinguish residual cancer from necroses and other residual tissues.

- The metabolic information obtained from MRSI may also allow an expanded assessment of tumor

46

aggressiveness and the attendant risk of disease progression.

- An attempt should be made to improve prostate cancer staging accuracy both prior to and after therapy by performing a combined high-resolution anatomic (MRI) and metabolic (MRSI) imaging exam. The five receiver coils is used (endorectal coil combined with four external coils) to acquire anatomic images with much higher resolution than previously possible, as well as to perform spectroscopic imaging.

- The endorectal coil provides the necessary sensitivity to focus on the prostate and surrounding structures.

- The pelvic phased-array (4 external coils) allows a large enough field-of-view to assess pelvic lymph nodes and bone for metastatic disease. However, one problem with using multiple surface coils is variability in image quality and subsequent interpretation. This is primarily due to the fact that image intensity dramatically decreases with distance from the surface coil.

- Computer processing has been developed to create uniform images that have greatly improved the ease of interpretation. Additionally, improved MR technology has allowed for reduction in the time required for MRI, making it more feasible to add MRSI to the staging examination.

Item:

I am reminded of a patient who called me one day for guidance and said that he wanted to undergo a radical prostatectomy for prostate cancer. I relayed to him that in my revised book, entitled, *New Guidelines For Surviving Prostate Cancer* I indicated "Don't rush to surgery." I also stated that if a patient is opting for surgery, I suggest (and I strongly made this recommendation) that he should first get a spectroscopic MRI (MRSI) to pinpoint the location of his tumor. The patient took my advice and requested his physician to give him a prescription for undergoing a MRSI diagnostic test. His physician refused because he did not want to display his ignorance about the test. Two weeks after the operation, the patient called me back and reported that his doctor indicated his disease was not a T2, but a T3 he had seminal vesicle invasion. I said to him, "The spectroscopic MRI would have imaged the seminal vesicle." Even if the test is an ongoing investigational study, the mere idea such a test has positive predicted value of 77% (sensitivity–83%, specificity–98%, and negative predicitve value–98%) for SV invasion should be taken into consideration.

Realizing the Accuracy of the MRSI

The most important parameters used when assessing any imaging modality are sensitivity, specificity, and positive predicted value. *Sensitivity* is the proportion of men with prostate cancer who have an abnormal imaging test. *Specificity* refers to the proportion of men who do not have prostate cancer and have a normal imaging test. *Positive predicted value* refers to the probability that an abnormal imaging test is due to prostate cancer. The addition of 3D-MRSI to MRI provides better detection and localization of prostate cancer alone. ROC analysis showed significantly (p ≤0.001) improved tumor localization for both readers when MRSI was added to MRI. High specificity (up to 91%) was obtained when both MRI and 3D–MRSI indicated cancer, whereas a positive result of either test provided high sensitivity (up to 95%). Additionally, the addition of MR spectroscopic imaging to MRI improves the diagnostic accuracy and decreases the interobserver variability of MRI in the diagnosis of extracapsular extension of prostate cancer. Adding MRSI to MRI for the more experienced reader improved accuracy (Az 0.86) over the use of MRI or MRSI alone. Adding MRSI to MRI for the less experienced reader improved accuracy (Az 0.75) to a level comparable to the more experienced MRI reader (Az 0.78).

Why did We Select This Diagnostic Technique?

There are several reasons why this diagnostic test was selected as the best technique for staging localized prostate cancer:

1. It has the highest degree of accuracy for localizing cancer within the prostate and assessing whether it has spread outside the gland.

2. The number of patients who are understaged or overstaged will be minimized.

3. The MRSI can distinguish metabolic differences between prostate cancer, normal tissue, and BPH better than any other technique.

4. The entire prostate can be evaluated in one study with excellent clarity.

5. The potential is unlimited.

How You May Use This Information

1. If your pathologic grade, clinical stage, and biochemical parameters (PSA, PAP) can pinpoint your disease at either end of the spectrum (definitely localized or definitely metastatic), you may not need an MRI/MRSI staging exam. However, for cancers that fall in between or for those patients who need a baseline for a less aggressive approach, additional local staging is important.

Don't undergo a radical prostatectomy before getting an MRI/MRSI to determine the exact location of your prostate cancer. If the results indicate your cancer has spread outside the gland, don't proceed with the surgery.

2. Don't have a CT scan or a bone scan if your PSA level is less than 10 ng/ml. Instead, get an MRSI as a reference point or baseline.

3. Monitor your disease after treatment with the MRSI.

4. Have an MRSI if you are undergoing any treatment for prostate cancer.

5. Don't be alarmed if your physician is not aware of the MRSI. This imaging test is relatively new, and doctors will need more time to learn about it.

Chapter 4

The Best Method for Conducting a Prostate Biopsy

5–Region Biopsy

Since the 1980's, the ability to diagnose prostate cancer has been enhanced significantly by the advent of the prostate specific antigen (PSA) test. By taking a PSA level and performing a digital rectal exam on an annual basis, physicians are now able to detect prostate cancer at an early stage (when it is confined to the prostate). Such early detection may represent the best chance for cure and for decreasing morbidity and mortality from this terrible disease. The sextant biopsy, which is usually guided by a transrectal ultrasound machine, has detected a large number of cases of prostate cancer. However, one research study has indicated that the sextant biopsy misses about 22 percent of the cancers. Many physicians have felt that six-tissue extractions of the prostate gland are not enough, and they have increased this figure to seven, eight, and even higher. Depending on the number of suspicious areas, one doctor may take as many as 18 samples from a patient.

At least one urologist uses magnetic resonance spectroscopic imaging (MRSI) to guide where he performed the biopsy of the patient for better coverage.

Urologists at the Bowman Gray School of Medicine of Wake Forest University at Winston-Salem, North Carolina, have discovered a technique known as the *5–region prostate biopsy*. It is superior to the sextant biopsy and represents, to this author, the best approach for conducting a prostate biopsy.

A study was conducted to determine if additional biopsies performed in areas of the prostate beyond those sampled by the sextant biopsy increased the detection of prostate cancer. A total of 119 patients underwent transrectal ultrasound-guided needle biopsy. In addition to sextant biopsies, cores were taken from the lateral and middle regions of the prostate gland. Pathological findings of the additional regions were analyzed and compared to these of the sextant biopsies. Of the 119 patients, 48 (40%) had prostate cancer. Of these 48 patients, 17 (35%) had cancer only in regions 1, 3, and 5 (right lateral, middle, and left lateral lobes). These tumors would have been missed had the sextant biopsy been used alone. (See figure 4-1.)

Figure 4-1 Posterior view of prostate gland as seen through the rectal wall. The 5-region biopsy is performed in this area.

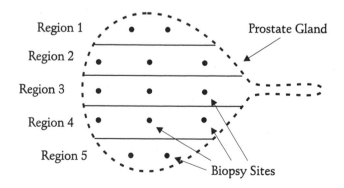

Preparation for the Biopsy

The first step to take in preparing for a needle biopsy of the prostate is to stop taking any medication that might interfere with the ability of the blood to clot. Then, two days prior to the biopsy, begin taking the antibiotic that your doctor has prescribed. (Generally, Cipro, Floxin, or Levaquin is prescribed.) If you have an artificial joint, such as an artificial hip, or a pacemaker, or other implanted device, additional or different antibiotics might be required. If you have a heart murmur or an abnormality of a heart valve, special arrangements for intravenous antibiotics will need to be made.

Prior to the biopsy, eat breakfast. Eat lunch if the biopsy is in the afternoon. Following the biopsy, you can resume your regular diet.

In the morning, use a Fleet's enema. If the biopsy is scheduled for early morning, it might be more convenient to use the enema the night before.

You need to be off any blood thinners or antiplatelet drugs for a sufficient period of time prior to the biopsy, so that your clotting is normal. If you take aspirin on a regular basis, stop it one to two weeks before undergoing the biopsy. If you have had a stroke or transient ischemic attack (TIA), it is not always safe to stop taking aspirin. In this case, alternative arrangements need to be made. Similarly, if you take Ticlid, discontinue it two weeks prior to the biopsy. Persantine (dipyridamole) should be stopped for two days and Coumadin (warfarin) for five days prior to a biopsy. For some patients, it will be necessary to receive intravenous heparin shortly after stopping the Coumadin. It is very important that before discontinuing Coumadin, you speak with the doctor who prescribed it. Finally, any nonsteroidal anti-inflammatory agents that you might take—such as Motrin, Advil, Nuprin, ibuprofen, Aleve, and Naprosyn—should be stopped two days prior to the biopsy.

However, it is all right to take Tylenol, Tylenol with codeine, or Percocet before the biopsy.

During the Biopsy

On the day of the biopsy, bring any medicines prescribed by your family doctor to the urologist's office. Generally, patients take two pills of Percocet (which is basically Tylenol with an opiate called oxycodone), and 5 mg of Valium (diazepan). After arriving in the office and checking that the biopsy will take place on schedule, take the sedative pills as prescribed. However, a wife was concerned because her husband was prescribed no medication. She goes on to say, "this made me want to cry. My husband, when he went for a biopsy early last year, was given no such sedation. When he went in for the procedure, he asked the doctor whether he would give him something. He was told he wouldn't need it. Well, when he left the doctor and came out to the waiting room, the look on his face was the look of a person who had been tortured. He had been through agony. To top it off, he was sent home with *no* pain medication. Thankfully, we had codeine in the house—he had to take it, he was in so much pain."

During the biopsy, you may feel pressure, as if you have to urinate. Some patients feel pressure as if they have to move their bowels. While a biopsy may be unpleasant, it is not painful, and it is easily tolerated by most patients. However, if the patient seems anxious, the urologist may give him a sedative. In situations where many samples are going to be extracted the biopsy is sometimes done in the hospital and the patient is put under anesthesia.

Transrectal ultrasound with an ultrasound-guided biopsy of the prostate is done in the urologist's office. You will be asked to lie on your left side on an exam table. An ultrasound probe, shaped like a finger, is covered with a latex condom that has been lubricated with water-soluble jelly, and is inserted through the anus into the rectum.

Using the probe, pictures of the prostate are obtained. The pictures show the size and dimensions of the prostate, the size and shape of the seminal vesicles, the condition of the capsule around the prostate, and any areas of abnormality within the prostate tissue. If, in the tissue near the rectal surface or on the lateral sides of the prostate, there is an area that transmits sound better than the surrounding tissue, it will appear darker. Such an area has a greater possibility of having prostate cancer than does adjacent tissue that has a higher ability to reflect sound and which would appear lighter in color.

To obtain the best views of the prostate, two ultrasound probes are generally used. The biopsy of the prostate is performed with guidance from a third ultrasound probe, which has more maneuverability for guiding the placement of the needle. This spring-loaded needle is placed within a guide pathway along the side of the ultrasound probe. The needle traverses the rectal wall and enters the prostate, driven by a spring, which makes the procedure very quick.

To thoroughly sample the prostate, the doctor will perform a sextant biopsy (six tissue extractions) and then will extract tissues from the right lateral, middle, and left lateral regions, for a total of 13 biopsies (see Figure 4-1). The tissues are subsequently sent to a pathologist to determine whether prostate cancer is present.

After the Biopsy

After the procedure, do not drive right away. Have someone else drive you home. After the biopsy a small percentage of patients may have some difficulty urinating. If this happens, call your doctor. He or she will probably insert a Foley catheter, a tube that passes through the urinary passageway of the penis and drains the bladder. It can be connected to a bag that is worn on the leg underneath trousers. Generally, after a few days of drainage, the catheter will be taken out, and normal urination will resume.

Although it is possible to have rectal bleeding after the biopsy, generally it clears up after a few of days.

There is usually some blood in the urine. The urine can be light red to pink for two or three days, and there may be a spot of blood at the start or finish of urination for a few weeks. A week after the biopsy, a small stringy clot may pass in the urinary stream, although the urine itself may be yellow.

Avoid any vigorous activity for the first couple of days after the biopsy, and avoid sexual activity for four or five days following the biopsy. Blood will be present in the ejaculate (semen) for two months. Do not be alarmed. If the blood in the ejaculate is dark red, this means it is old, and you may continue with sexual activity. If the blood is very bright red, wait another week before engaging in sexual activity. It is possible that a biopsy might stir up an old prostate infection or create a new urinary tract or prostate infection. However, the likelihood of these events is low.

Limitations of the Prostate Biopsy

Biopsies have certain limitations, as follows:

1. Sometimes, cancer is present, but the biopsy needle misses it. Known as a *sampling error* this occurs about 15 percent of the time. If a patient's biopsy is negative, but his DRE and PSA test indicate cancer, he should return to the physician's office in three months for a follow-up.

2. At times, the biopsy may not reveal the full extent of the cancer. The tissues extracted from the prostate may show only a small amount of the tumor when there is actually much more.

3. The biopsy may be uncomfortable or painful for some men. Some physicians give the patient a local sedative.

4. The biopsy itself may spread the cancer; like all surgical procedures, it poses a risk.

5. The biopsy may transfer germs from the rectum into the prostate. However, this is rare, as most men are instructed to have an enema before the biopsy and to take antibiotics before and after it.

6. The biopsy may cause the prostate to swell which may lead to difficulty in urinating.

7. A patient with a grade III PIN is usually asked to revisit the office of the urologist for a repeat biopsy.

Purposes of the Biopsy

Biopsies have several purposes:

1. Primarily, the biopsy is used to determine a patient's stage and Gleason score, critical elements in predicting the aggressiveness of his disease.

2. It is also used to perform a DNA ploidy analysis- that is, to determine if the tumor is diploid, tetraploid, or aneuploid.

3. If your doctor suspects disease in your seminal-vesicles, a biopsy is sometimes necessary to rule out progression of cancer before treatment. This is most likely to be beneficial to men with bulky, higher-grade tumors. Among 67 men who underwent radical prostatectomy for clinically localized prostate cancer, Vallancien and coworkers determined that seminal-vesicle biopsy detected 61 percent of those men with seminal-vesicle invasion with no false-positive biopsies. They recommended seminal-vesicle biopsy in all men

with localized prostate cancer and a PSA level of less than 10 ng/ml.

4. Branches of the neurovascular bundles enter the prostate on the posterior lateral surface. Prostate cancer frequently penetrates the capsule of the prostate, the perineural space invasion. Bastacky and colleagues evaluated the findings of perineural-invasion needle biopsies as a prediction of capsular penetration among 302 men with stage 2 prostate cancer who underwent surgery. Perineural invasion was seen in 20 percent of pretreatment needle biopsies.

5. Five-region biopsy is taken from several different areas of the prostate to get a good representative sampling of the entire gland, including the sextant biopsy as described by Hodge et al. including two biopsies from each lateral aspect of the gland and three from the middle of the prostate. A total of at least 13 biopsies per patient.

6. Some patients run a fever after a biopsy.

Other Important Information About Biopsies

Patients should be aware of the following:

Different Types of Cancer

Several types of cancer can occur in the body. Cancer of muscles, bones, and supporting tissues are *sarcomas,* which are very rare. Cancers of the blood and lymphatic systems are known as *leukemias* or *lymphomas.* Cancer of protective linings (coverings of organs such as the inside of the mouth) or of the skin are frequently *squamous* cancers. Cancers arising from glands that absorb or secrete fluids are called *adenocarcinomas.* The cancers frequently arise in the pancreas, colon, rectum, and lower esophagus and other digestive organs, as well as in the lung and prostate.

The Type of Cancer Usually Found in the Prostate

Prostate cancer, or *prostatic adenocarcinoma*, is cancer of the glands in the prostate that secrete fluid that makes up most of the semen.

How The Pathologist Identifies Cancer

The pathologist looks for unusual cells, especially ones where the nucleus becomes relatively large compared with the cytoplasm. (The nucleus is where DNA, the Cell's blueprint, is kept.) You can think of this as the yolk and the white of an egg. Cancer cells reproduce at a very high rate, and so the nucleus is busy turning out lots of copies of the DNA. If the nucleus were an egg yolk, it would become very large compared to the white. This distortion of the nuclear: cytoplasmic ratio is characteristic of cancer cells.

In addition, because prostate cells form glands which are separated by muscle and supporting tissue layers, the pathologist looks for distortions of gland formation. Bizarre or disorganized glands, formation of "glands in glands" ("cribriform gland formation"), and back-to-back glands without intervening tissue are all signs of cancer. The diagnostic finding of cancer, however, is the presence of cells or groups of cells invading beyond their natural borders into other areas of the prostate gland.

*This information comes from the website of Radiotherapy Clinics of Georgia.

Why We Chose This Procedure

We chose the 5–region biopsy as the best option for the following reasons:

1. It has discovered 37 percent more cancer in patients than has standard biopsies.

2. It minimizes the number of "false claims."

3. It significantly increases the chance of detecting prostate cancer on the first try.

4. Finding the cancer at the earliest stage gives the patient more options for treatment.

How You May Use This Information

To save yourself time, anxiety, and cost, consider the following:

1. If your doctor is unaware of the 5-region biopsy, share this chapter with him or her.

2. If your urologist fails to detect prostate cancer using a sextant biopsy, ask him or her to perform a 5-region biopsy three months after the first try.

3. Multicolor transrectal ultrasound will usually pick up a greater number of suspicious spots than will a black-and-white ultrasound.

Chapter 5

THE BEST METHOD FOR APPLYING EXTERNAL BEAM RADIATION TO PROSTATE CANCER

External Beam Radiation Plus Zoladex

There seems to be little agreement about which treatment for prostate cancer should be given first. There are strong proponents of radical prostatectomy and equally dogmatic supporters of external beam radiation. Some urologists have been known to suggest radiation when surgery is no longer warranted.

For a prostate cancer patient who has decided to undergo radiation, there are numerous decisions to be made. Should he receive proton beam, neutrons, or photon beam? Should he receive combination hormonal therapy before, during, or after radiation? Should he get the combining therapy radiation field or the conventional radiation field? It is inappropriate to talk generically about the effectiveness of radiation when each of the above questions must be carefully considered. The decisions that are made will determine to a great extent, treatment outcome.

Methods for Improving External Beam Radiation Through Dose Escalation

Over the years, several attempts have been made to improve external beam radiation. This chapter will discuss those attempts made to improve the effectiveness of external radiation and why the combined modality treatment using external beam radiation and Zoladex are identified as the "best" external bean radiation treatment for prostate cancer.

Studies have shown that the size of the dose delivered to the patient is related to some extent, on the effectiveness of the treatment. For example, Perez and colleagues reported that 38 percent of patients with stage C disease had local recurrence with doses of fewer than 60 Gy, compared to 20 percent of patients with dosages of 60 to 70 Gy and 12 percent for patients who received more than 70 Gy. Similar forms exist from the patterns of case studies group for 1,348 stage B and C patients.

The actual 5-year local recurrence rate for stage C patients was 37 percent for doses of less than 60 Gy; 36 percent for 60 Gy; 28 percent for 65 to 69 Gy; and 19 percent for more than 70 Gy. Dose escalation seems justified according to these studies. However, the side effects of external beam radiation restrict attempts to increase the dose above 70 Gy. When using photon beam radiation, rectal bleeding increases from 12 to 20 percent. Although there are few clinical data attesting to the relationship of volume to complications for either rectum or bladder, there are decreased side effects with conformal radiation. One study, which included 41 patients, has suggested that there is a dose-volume relationship for rectal bleeding. A high probability of complications ranged between 60 CGE (cobalt grey equivalent) delivered to 70 percent of the anterior rectal wall and 75 CGE to 30 percent. Another problem inherent in radiation sensitivity is that it may vary between patients and tests. To detect sensitive patients populations using this protocol would be useful in deleting patients from external beam radiation, particularly those undergoing dose-escalation techniques.

Conformal Radiation

Conformal radiation is getting a great deal of attention in the United States. In fact, if a medical center performing external beam radiation on prostate cancer patients does not use this approach, it is said to behind the times. Conformal radiation employs several criteria to improve external beam radiation, including accurate patient positioning; computed tomography (CT) planning with three-dimensional reconstruction of volumes; clear definition of treatment margins; and meticulous verification procedures of the shaped fields produced by customized shaped blocks or multileaf collimation.

Although multiple planar and complex noncoplanar beam orientation are an improvement over the more simple arrangements in terms of more moderate degrees of dose escalation, there has not been any significant improvement. The amount of normal tissue treated to the 90 percent isodose may be decreased by 42 percent, with 46 and 41 percent reductions in the volumes of bowel and bladder, respectively. According to studies reported by three North American groups using careful planning and immobilization techniques, doses of 75 Gy have been well tolerated, and currently doses in excess of 80 Gy are being delivered.

Precision Dosing a Reality With Intensity Modulated Radiation Therapy

Recently, an attempt has been made to improve on conventional conformal radiation. Advances in three fields–

imaging, medical physics, and computer technology–have led to the development of a radiation therapy modality that may represent a significant breakthrough in cancer treatment.

"Intensity modulated radiation therapy (IMRT) is the most sophisticated form of computer-delivered radiation therapy currently available," said David E. Wazer, MD, director of the Radiation Oncology Center of the New England Medical Center, which pioneered the technique.

IMRT is not just an improvement on state-of-the-art radiation therapy, but rather it offers a complete change in the way in which radiation therapy is administered.

IMRT is a three-dimensional conformal radiation treatment that uses a powerful computer model to plan therapy and a multileaf intensity-modulated collimator (MIMic) to deliver highly focused radiation doses while causing minimal damage to surrounding tissue.

Dr. Engler, a physicist-in-chief at the Radiation Oncology Center, maintains that, in effect, all radiation therapy is conformal. "Obviously, from the time the first physicians aimed an X-ray tube at a cancer, they wanted the dose to conform to the target." According to Engler, unlike conventional 3D-conformal radiation therapy (3D-CRT), IMRT treatment decisions are based on complex mathematical modes, resulting in a level of precision previously unattainable.

The Planning Phase

In planning treatment with IMRT, a series of 40 to 80 CT images are obtained and sent to the planning computer where radiation oncology personnel delineate the targets and the sensitive surrounding normal tissues. The clinician then determines the optimal dosage for the tumor site and the maximum tolerated dosages for the surrounding normal organs and tissues. This allows for external radiation dosage that spares normal tissues.

"In a prostate cancer patient, for example, the physician can tell the computer the maximum tolerated dose for the rectum, the bladder, the heads of the femurs, and so forth," Dr. Engler said. "In a brain tumor patient, the system forces the physician to quantify the relative importance of, say, the auditory nerve versus the optic nerve."

Once all the data are entered, the IMRT software simulates the radiation physics for the desired doses, using mathematical models to search for the plan that best satisfies the physician's multifaceted prescription. The plan typically includes "an astronomical number of beam patterns, providing dynamic, optimized, intensity-modulated 3D radiation therapy," Dr. Engler said.

The data for the optimal plan are then transferred to a disk, which is inserted into the multileaf intensity-modulated collimater (MIMic) controller on the accelerator for delivery of the treatment plan.

As the MIMic rotates around the patient, it constantly measures the beam angle and adjusts the small vanes that shape the beam. Thus, the field shape and intensity of the beam are continuously varied so as to mold the radiation beam to the target and modulate the intensity of the radiation across the target.

In contrast, with conventional 3D-CRT, the radiotherapist is aiming at a silhouette of the target, and you're treating normal tissues in front of and behind that silhouette in a somewhat arbitrary fashion. "IMRT technology is aimed at minimizing the dose to these tissues in front of and behind the target in a very systematic manner with intensity modulation."

Typically, the prescription dose is about 85 percent of the maximum dose. "The whole point of this system is that it creates a very sharp falloff of dose right around the target," Dr. Engler said.

Prostate cancer is now being treated using IMRT. The system is allowing radiotherapists to cut down the dosages to the rectum and bladder by about 50 percent. Several years of follow-up will be necessary to determine if the technique does indeed produce fewer complications.

Particle Beam Radiation

Probably the best method of improving radiation dose distribution using external beam treatment is the use of particle therapy with protons

Neutron beam radiation is no better than photon beam radiation, but it does have a higher linear energy transfer, which may produce an increased efficacy against certain radio-resistant tumors. Studies in stage C and D have shown that mixed neutron-photon external beam radiation randomized study has shown that neutron therapy improves local central and normalizes PSA levels in comparison with photon beam therapy. Clinical or biochemical failure occurred in 32 percent and 45 percent of patients in the photon arm compared with 11 percent and 17 percent in the neutron arm. However, at the expense of increased grade 3 complications (11% vs. 30%), there was a strong indication that the use of beam shaping using multileaf collimation (MLC) reduces late radiation toxicity. In the subgroup of patients treated at the University of Washington using an MLC, no excess side effects were observed, although improvements in local control were maintained. However, the technology to produce particle beam therapy is very expensive, and unless clinical trials show good results, it is unlikely that these techniques will gain wide acceptance.

Particle beam therapy has an advantage over photon beam radiation because it distributes energy over a small area. It allows a high dose to be provided to the target area with a sharp falloff in dose to surrounding tissues. In Massachusetts, a randomized trial has demonstrated a small improvement in the rate of local control rate (77% vs. 60% at 8 years), particularly for poorly differentiated tumors;

this has produced important information on dose-volume relationships for complications. The rate of incidental rectal bleeding increased when doses were increased from 67.2 Gy to 75.6 CGE. At the higher dose level, 20 percent of the patients had this complication 18 less than 40 percent of the anterior rectal wall was treated compared with 72 percent of patients when more than 40 percent received radiation. A small advantage exists for proton beam therapy within two opposing fields, compared with three- or six-field photon beam radiation. About one-third of cases had benefits from a proton beam plan. Any advantage in the remaining patients was limited because of the need to include the anterior rectal wall in the target area; thus, the real advantages of proton beam radiation may be limited to prostate cancer.

Combined-Modality Treatment Using Hormones and Radiation

Combining combination hormonal therapy (CHT) and external beam radiation (EBR) has two advantages. First, combined-modality treatment may lead to increased tumor kill, because CHT probably causes apoptosis and EBR induces mitotic cell death. Secondly, initial shrinkage of the prostate and prostate cancer can lead to a beneficial modification of the radiation treatment area. Reducing the radiation treatment volume may positively affect the therapeutic ratio, either by reducing radiation aftereffects for a standard radiation dose or by permitting dose escalation; this should increase tumor control while maintaining acceptable levels of radiation complications. In addition to these potential benefits, CHT may have advantages in the therapeutic result that is achieved by one modality treating disease missed by the other.

Researchers at the Royal Marsden Hospital, using three to six months of initial luteinizing hormone-releasing hormone (LHRH) analog treatment, have demonstrated a 50 percent reduction in the prostate-gland volume and an associated 40 percent potential reduction in external beam radiation treatment volume. Results indicated that 70 percent of the patients with a bulky stage T_2 to T_4 prostate cancer remained in biochemical remission 18 months after treatment. A randomized study has been undertaken by the RTOG in North America. A total of 457 men with bulky stage B2/C prostate cancer were randomly selected to receive Zoladex and Eulexin for two months before and during external beam radiation, or to receive external beam radiation alone. With a median potential follow-up of 4.5 years, the incidence of local progression over 5 years was 46 percent for the combined-modality treatment compared with 71 percent for external beam radiation alone. The 5-year incidence rates of distant metastases were 34 and 41 percent, respectively. Biochemical progression-free survival rates indicated an advantage with the combined-modality group, with 36 percent progression-free at 5 years compared with 15 percent in patients treated with external beam radiation alone.

The benefit of combined-modality treatment using CHT and EBR has been shown in breast cancer. But only recently has it been shown to be effective in prostate cancer.

The New England Journal of Medicine, (July 31, 1997, Vol. 337, No. 5) published a study by Michael Bolla, M.D., et al. on prostate cancer patients treated with radiotherapy and goserelin. From 1987 to 1995, a total of 415 patients with locally advanced prostate cancer were randomly assigned to receive external beam radiation (photon-beam) alone or with Zoladex. The group of patients had a median age of 71 years (range: 51 to 80). Patients in the two groups receive 50 Gy of radiation to the pelvis over a period of 5 weeks, and an additional 20 Gy over an additional 2 weeks as a boost. Patients in the combined-treatment group received 3.6 mg of Zoladex every 4 weeks starting on the day of radiation, continuing the LHRH agonist for 3 years. These patients also received 150 mg (orally) of cyproterane acetate daily during the first month of treatment in order to stop the rise of testosterone associated with Zoladex.

The test data were available for analysis on 401 patients. The median follow-up was 45 months. Overall survival rates for 5 years, estimated by the Kaplan-Meyer calculation, were 79 percent in the combined-treatment group and 62 percent in the external beam radiation group. As a result, the group receiving EBR plus the Zoladex experienced a 17 percent increase over the group undergoing EBR alone.

Why We Selected This Option

We selected EBR combined with CHT for the following reasons:

1. It was based on a clinical study.

2. It proved Dr. Thomas Stamey's theory that undergoing CHT before, during, and after external beam radiation with hormone therapy improves overall survival.

How You May Use This Information

1. Do not undergo external beam radiation without CHT.

2. If your radiologist wants to irradiate you without also prescribing CHT, ask for proof that his or her protocol is superior to that presented in the *New England Journal of Medicine* July 31, 1997, Vol. 337, No. 5.

Chapter 6

The Best Complementary Therapy for Prostate Cancer Patients

PC SPES

Approximately 70 percent of all patients diagnosed with prostate cancer will develop metastatic disease at some time in the course of their illness. Currently, hormone-refractory metastatic prostate cancer is not curable. As a result, treatment for this condition has been predominately focused on palliating symptoms, such as bone pain.

Current treatments for newly diagnosed prostate cancer patients include watchful waiting, radical prostatectomy, external beam radiation, brachytherapy, cryosurgery, hyperthermia, and hormonal therapy. However, once the disease has escaped the capsule of the prostate gland, there is little chance of cure. Once the disease has metastasized, the patient is usually given hormonal therapy consisting of an LHRH agonist (such as Lupron) with or without an antiandrogen (such as Casadex). However, only 80 percent of patients respond to hormone treatment and then only for a median time of 2 years. Sooner or later, most patients undergoing hormone therapy will reach a hormone-refractory state, and hormones will no longer palliate their disease. In the best of cases, a mere 8 to 10 percent of patients on hormones survive 10 years or more.

Unfortunately, the only other therapy available for hormone-refractory patients is chemotherapy, which has a variety of side effects and can only keep patients alive for a limited time.

A multitude of salvage regimens for hormone-refractory patients are under investigation; however, clinical trials have not yet reported any significant success.

A complementary therapy, an herbal formula known as PC SPES, has received widespread attention among prostate cancer patients. It is considered the best treatment for hormone-refractory patients because it is the only one that seems to induce apoptosis (cell death) and stimulate the immune system.

A German study, as well as many anecdotal reports, supports the author's claim that PC SPES is the "best" and only treatment for hormone-refractory disease. The study was conducted by Bernd L. Pfeifer, M.D., and colleagues at the Division of Urology and Department of Anesthesiology, University of Kentucky, and Department of Urology, Allgemeines Krankenhaus Celle, Germany. Us Too International conducted a survey among their members taking PC SPES, and the results also support my claim.

Sixteen men treated for metastatic prostate cancer with either an orchiectomy (castration) or an LHRH agonist with or without an antiandrogen, entered into a clinical trial to evaluate the effects of PC SPES. After failing hormone therapy, these patients took three capsules of PC SPES (960 mg) three times daily for 5 months. Hormonal therapy was continued throughout the trial to avoid the effects of antiandrogen withdrawal.

Results of the study indicated that patients taking PC SPES had a significant improvement in the quality of life and in reduction of pain, and they had a dramatic decrease in their PSA levels. A total of 81 percent of patients achieved a greater than 50 percent decline in their PSA level (as compared to their pre- PC SPES level). Improved quality of life was reported by 94 percent of the patients. The number of bone lesions declined by about 65 percent, thus indicating the retardation of prostate cancer cell growth.

Herbs for Healing

Herbs can be found almost everywhere. They are as near to us as the thyme in our spice racks or the grass on our lawns. Herbal medicines, which have been used for thousands of years, are currently receiving a great deal of interest from physicians and researchers.

Plants have always been humanity's closest companion. Although we could survive without animals, we could not survive without plants. They are an essential part of our existence. In addition to being a major source of food, clothing, shelter, and fuel, plants also provide the very air that we breathe. Plants literally capture the energy of the sun, transforming sunlight into the food used to sustain their life and growth. As a by-product of this photosynthesis—transformation of light into energy—plants emit the very oxygen that we breathe.

In addition to keeping the atmosphere rich with oxygen, many plants have therapeutic properties that can be used to heal prostate cancer. PC SPES is made from a unique blend of these plants.

Herbs Enhance the Immune System

Except for the sympathetic nervous system, perhaps no other system in the human body is better suited to herbal compounds than the immune system. In order to nurture a healthy body (or to improve an unhealthy one), the immune system must be constantly ready to search for and eliminate antigens or foreign substances.

It is imperative that you do all you can to strengthen and keep your immune system strong, while taking great care not to overstimulate it, as too many white blood cells can be just as harmful as too few. Certain herbal medicines have the potential to normalize and balance the immune system. In addition, in the event of an infection, such medicines can be used to intensify the immune system's response. In the event of an overactive immune system— for example, an allergic reaction—herbal medicine can also be applied.

Numerous studies have shown that some of the most powerful immune-system boosters come from specific healing herbs. Some of these plants are *adaptogens*, which strengthen and normalize the nervous and hormonal systems, thereby helping us to adapt to the multitude of stresses that we are exposed to. Some herbs also contain antioxidant complements, which can delay the cellular aging process and enhance the immune system as well. Others contain immunosaturating polysaccharides, which help the immune system to combat foreign invaders, such as bacteria and viruses, and have the potential to battle cancer. They are also useful in relieving the side effects of certain conventional treatments for prostate cancer, such as chemotherapy and radiation. Other herbs are powerful tonics that strengthen the immune system at a much deeper level. These herbs support the functions of T cells, activate macrophages, and suppress cancer growth.

Scientists and medical doctors have worked for years to identify the most appropriate blend of herbs with which to treat certain diseases and illnesses. As a result of these studies, the formula used to produce PC SPES was developed by chemist Sophie Chen, Ph.D., and her colleagues, Allan

Wang, M.D., and Hui Fu Wang, M.D., who integrated modern science and ancient wisdom.

What is PC SPES?

PC SPES, a unique blend of herbs contains specific properties that enhance the immune system. It provides multiple benefits to prostate cancer patients. The very name of the product is indicative of the hope that it offers: *PC* stands for *prostate cancer* and *spes* is Latin for *hope*. PC SPES is meant to help prostate cancer patients either by saving their lives or, by extending their survival time.

PC SPES contains only certified organic herbal extracts harvested at the best time and at specific geographical locations to insure maximum potency and quality. The dried herbs are processed and refined according to proprietary technology in order to assure their effectiveness and safety.

Following are the eight herbs that make up PC SPES:

- *Isatis indigotica* (da quing ye) is a Chinese herb that contains beta-sitosterol, a phytosterol. Phytosterols are constituents of legumes and other plants. They are structurally similar to cholesterol. Oral administration of plant sterols bind to cholesterol and reduce its absorption from the gastrointestinal tract. Oral administration of beta-sitosterol is known to reduce tumor size in tumor-bearing animals.

- *Glycyrrhiza glabra* and *Glycyrrhiza uralensis* (gan cao) are saponin-containing Chinese herbs. Glycyrrhiza is used in traditional herbal medicine called SKT (Shakuyaku-Kanzo-To). The Kanzo portion contains glycyrrhiza root along with the licoflavone putresin. These substances bind cholesterol and bile acids and have surfactant properties. There is evidence that saponins stimulate the immune system and inhibit the expression of Epstein-Barr virus. Saponins possess invitro antitumor activities. Glycyrrhiza also contains quercetin, which has been found in many other herbs and in fruits, and has been demonstrated to have antitumor effects. Glycyrrhiza lowers serum testosterone levels and correspondingly increases estrogen levels through stimulation or induction of 17-B-hydroxysteroid dehydrogenase and the aromatase enzyme. Glycyrrhiza is metabolically converted to glycyrrhetic acid (GA) when incubated invitro with adrenal gland cells. GA has been shown to increase DHEA production.

- *Panax pseudo-ginseng* (san qi) contains dammarane-type saponins that are adaptagenic (nonspecific antistress, homeostatis-inducing properties). It is purported to enhance immunity by stimulating natural-killer cells.

- *Ganoderma lucidum* (ling zhi) is a Chinese herb containing high molecular weight polysaccharide compounds that are obtained by water extraction. The extracts markedly inhibited growth of sarcoma 180 cells implanted into mice, and injections of a water solution of the extracts into mice bearing lung carcinoma cells increased life spans up to 195 percent.

- *Scutellaria baicalensis* (huang qin) is a Chinese herb that has been shown invitro to inhibit the growth of sarcoma 180, sarcoma 37, and cervical cancer cells. Also, this herb inhibits platelet aggregation and histamine release invitro. In addition, baicalein inhibits tumor-cell proliferation and induces apoptosis invitro. It has been shown to stimulate the immune system in vivo and to possess antibacterial effects that may alter the flora of the gastrointestinal tract.

- *Dendranthema* (Chrysanthemum) *morifolium Tzvel* is a lesser-known Chinese herb with unspecified biologic effects.

- *Rabdosia rebescens* is a Chinese herb with multiple antitumor and analgesic properties. Invitro, it inhibits hela cells, Ehrlich ascites cells, sarcoma 180 cells, hepatoma cells, cervical carcinoma U14 cells (mice), Walker 256 carcinosarcoma cells, and reticular carcinoma cells. Analgesic and anti-anorexigenic properties have been observed in hepatoma patients taking this herb. Increased survival time and reduced side effects as a result of antineoplastic treatment has been noted in patients with esophageal carcinoma.

- saw palmetto (*Serenoa repens*) is an herb that decreases the bioavailability of testosterone in vivo and also inhibits eicosanoid production. It has been shown to be as equally effective as the 5a-reductase inhibitor finasteride in the treatment of benign prostatic hyperplasia. Although saw palmetto is said to possess effects similar to 5a-reductase inhibitors, recent studies failed to demonstrate significant declines in dihydrotestosterone levels in treated patients.

Based on their pharmacological activities, these eight herbs are divided into five categories:

1. immune-stimulating

2. antitumor

3. antiviral

4. anti-inflammatory

5. anti-benign prostate hyperplasia

Properties of PC SPES

Some of the properties of PC SPES follow:

- It neutralizes free radicals through antioxidant action.

- It lowers or raises red blood cell count depending on need.

- It lowers or raises white blood cell count depending on need.

- It is nontoxic compared to most conventional drugs.

- It has a distinct antitoxic action against a wide range of toxins.

- It induces cancer-cell death.

- It is good for the central nervous system.

- It suppresses the cancer gene bcl-6 and enhances the immune system.

- It suppresses androgen receptors.

- It changes the cancer-cell growth cycle.

Side Effects

Patients taking PC SPES may or may not experience side effects, depending on their health, other drugs they are taking, and the stage of their disease.

Possible side effects of PC PES include:

Nipple soreness and breast enlargement.

These are also side effects of hormone therapy. However, PC SPES does not cause the other side effects associated with hormone therapy, such as memory loss, hot flashes, osteoporosis, and depression. If this particular side effect becomes too difficult for you to bear, the dosage of PC SPES can be reduced. Another option is to apply progesterone cream to the breast.

Decline in libido.

Softening of the stool, or diarrhea.

If this condition exists, the patient should ask the doctor to prescribe either Immodium or Lomotil, or the patient may decrease the dosage of PC SPES.

Blood clot.

Two to 5 percent of patients taking large dosages (six to nine capsules daily) of PC SPES develop a blood clot in the leg causing swelling or pain. However, it remains to be proven that PC SPES actually causes blood clots to develop. Most men who have prostate cancer are at risk of developing clots whether or not they take PC SPES.

When a blood clot breaks loose, it can travel to the lung, causing chest pain or a pulmonary embolism. Sometimes a leg clot travels to the lung and causes a heart attack.

To avoid a blood clot, patients should take an aspirin a day or Coumadin. Also effective is 2,000 mg of aged garlic, 400 IU of vitamin E three times a day, and 1 to 2 capsules of Ginko Biloba. If you should develop a clot in the leg, take a blood thinner such as heparin. Once heparin has controlled the blood clot, switch to warfarin. Other drugs, called low molecular weight heparins, appear to be more effective and much safer than heparin or warfarin. Wearing support stockings can lessen the pain caused by a blood clot in the leg.

Safety

PC SPES should be stored in a cool, dry place, out of the reach of children.

PC SPES does not interfere with conventional treatments, and it can be ingested prior to, during, or after therapy. PC SPES has also been found to be beneficial to patients who are undergoing conventional treatments. If you have an infection, the effectiveness of PC SPES will be reduced until the infection has completely cleared.

Don't Rely on PC SPES Alone

Although PC SPES produces good to excellent results for prostate cancer patients, it should not be used alone. Instead, it should be taken in combination with a plan for good health. Always remember that your health depends on the harmonious interaction of all the components the body uses to recognize and destroy disease microorganisms. A plethora of evidence demonstrates that the use of herbs, along with proper eating habits, regular exercise, adequate sleep, and other proper health practices can strengthen the immune system to fight diseases.

Limitations

The effectiveness of PC SPES will be reduced when:

1. You have a cold.

2. You have an infection.

3. You have the flu.

4. You are on steroids.

5. You are experiencing physical stress, such as that caused by surgery, wounds, or injuries.

When the body is facing a foreign invasion (such as bacteria or a virus), the immune system will deal with the invasion first. The effect of PC SPES on the immune system thus becomes a secondary action to its response to the invasion.

PC SPES, PSA Level, and Tumor Size

Is it possible for PC SPES to decrease a patient's PSA level, yet not reduce the tumor? Many prostate cancer patients have this question. Dr. Abraham Mittelman, one of the physicians conducting a pilot study of PC SPES, has indicated that some patients had a notable decrease in their PSA levels but only a small decrease in the size of their tumors. However, a very large number of patients experienced a marked decrease in both PSA level and tumor size.

Laboratory experiments have shown that PC SPES can effectively kill cancer cells but does not affect normal white blood cells. It has also been shown that the reason the PSA level in a cancer cell decreases is because androgen receptors on the cell surface are suppressed, thus inactivating the PSA gene, which, in turn, induces cancer-cell death.

To understand why PC SPES can lower a patient's PSA level without dramatically affecting his tumor, it is important to understand how PC SPES works. PC SPES is a dietary supplement designed to enhance the body's immune system. Unfortunately, a prostate cancer patient's immune system can become very debilitated as a result of his overall health, the progression of the disease, or the effects of chemotherapy. When this occurs, no therapy can restore the immune system in a short time, no matter how healthy the patient appears to be. This condition is known as *immune-refractory disease*. In some patients, PC SPES still attempts to fight the prostate cancer. The supplement decreases the PSA level, but it does little to affect the tumor.

Although it is possible for PC SPES to decrease a patient's PSA level without reducing his tumor, the author has encountered far more instances where the treatment has done both. For example, one patient with a PSA level of 40.01 ng/ml took 2,700 mg of PC SPES for a little more than 2 months. His PSA dropped to 3.5. A posttreatment Prosta-Scint scan was compared to a pretreatment scan, and the pathologist reported "a marked interval regression of the disease." Another patient indicated that he had an RT-PCR PSA test to confirm the effect of PC SPES on his tumor. The result showed no evidence of the disease in the patient's body. Another man had before and after treatment ProstaScint scans. Again, the results indicated that after the patient had taken PC SPES, no evidence of the disease remained.

Evaluating The Effects of PC SPES

The *International Journal of Oncology* (13:0-00, 1998) reported that proliferation of Mutu I cells was inhibited by a 3- to 7-day incubation with ethanolic extracts of PC SPES with concurrent induction of apoptosis. Dr. Sophie Chen, the developer of PC SPES, says that it contains concentrated phytochemicals including flavonoids, alkanoids, polysaccharides, amino acids, and trace elements such as selenium, calcium, magnesium, zinc, and copper, which down-regulates the b/2 gene and induces cancer cell death. All these compounds have known pharmacological effects on cancer cells. Laboratory research has found that PC SPES can modulate the cancer-cell cycle and slow cancer cell growth; at the same time, it kills cancer cells by suppressing the cancer gene bcl-6, suppressing androgen receptors, and inactivating the PSA gene. It also effects b/2, b/6 gene, and androgen receptor. These are factors to suppress prostate cancer; therefore, PC SPES is not causing a decrease in the PSA.

In order to monitor their disease while taking PC SPES, patients should get a baseline image of their condition prior to beginning PC SPES. After about 6 months, they should get the same image for comparative analysis. Patients could use the MRSI to monitor their disease before and after treatment and to analyze the results. Some patients have reported some excellent comparisons using the prostaScint scan.

Dose Sensitivity

Patients taking PC SPES should be mindful of the following:

1. PC SPES is extremely dose-sensitive. BotanicLab recommends a starting dose of 6 capsules a day and appears to advise against anything greater than 12 per day.

2. There appears to be a "threshold" dosage; at this dose, a patient can expect his PSA level to fall, but below this dose, it will continue to rise, though more slowly than before. This threshold dosage can differ from patient to patient and depends on the stage.

3. At the threshold dosage, a patient can expect his PSA to drop quite rapidly the first month, less dramatically the second, still less dramatically the third, and so on, until it levels off at some number (it may actually continue to fall, but very slowly). This leveling-off point may be very low (below 0.1) or quite high (e.g., over 30). If, after this leveling-off occurs, the dosage is increased by even one capsule daily, the PSA will again fall more rapidly and will level off at a lower number.

4. Consistency is important in using PC SPES. Dosage should be kept constant. Doses must not be

missed. PC SPES is more effective when taken throughout the day. If you are taking six capsules per day, then two capsules three times a day is probably more effective than three taken twice a day, and so on.

5. When a patient stops taking PC SPES before his PSA level has "stabilized" for a long time at a very low level, the result is quite predictable: there is a sudden upsurge in PSA.

Clinical Trial

An ongoing clinical trial being conducted by E. J. Small, M.D., has reported some interesting findings on PC SPES. Patients received nine capsules a day of PC SPES. Two groups of prostate cancer patients were treated: (1) hormone-naïve (HN) patients demonstrating disease progression in the setting of normal testosterone levels, and (2) androgen-independent (AI) patients demonstrating disease progression in the setting of anorchid testosterone levels and after antiandrogen withdrawal. A total of 66 patients (32 HN, 34 AI) took PC SPES. Twenty-seven of the 32 hormone-naïve patients were evaluable; all of them had a PSA decline of more than 50 percent. Testosterone levels fell to anorchid levels after one month in 22 of the 27 (81%). Of the 34 androgen-independent patients, 19 (56%) had a PSA decline of over 50 percent. To date, toxicity has consisted of breast tenderness and enlargement in 82 percent of patients, and nausea and/or diarrhea in 39 percent. A single patient with advanced androgen independence had a pulmonary embolism. A total of 52 percent of patients with previous normal testosterone levels lost libido, and 33 percent became impotent. PC SPES is an effective agent in the treatment of hormone-naive PSA, but also is effective in patients with androgen-independent prostate cancer. Toxicity is manageable. Objective responses, time to progression, overall survival, and long-term toxicity remain under study.

Another Phase II clinical trial was recently completed but we are not at liberty to present it in detail before it is published in a scientific journal. The study involved 15 hormonal-refractory patients. The results indicated that 94 percent had an improvement in quality of life, more than 80 percent of the patients had a more than 50 percent decrease in their PSA, and more than 60 percent of the patients had relief of pain.

Why We Selected This Therapy

There are several reasons why we selected PC SPES as the best complementary therapy.

1. After a person becomes resistant to hormonal therapy, PC SPES is the only treatment available other than chemotherapy. Chemotherapy offers patients a limited survival time, and it kills healthy cells along with cancer cells, resulting in eventual death.

2. PC SPES might prevent or delay a recurrence of prostate cancer. However, additional studies are needed.

3. PC SPES might lengthen the survival time of prostate cancer patients by delaying the use of chemotherapy.

4. PC SPES can decrease tumor burden, thereby inhibiting the growth of prostate cancer.

5. PC SPES is an alternative treatment when combination hormone therapy is no longer effective.

6. PC SPES is an effective dietary supplement used to maintain patients on watchful waiting.

7. It is effective as an adjunct treatment either before, during, or after conventional treatment.

8. Two phase II clinical trials have proved that PC SPES is an effective treatment for prostate cancer.

How You May Use This Information

In order to make effective use of this information, consider the following:

1. While patients are encouraged to use PC SPES during watchful waiting, they should be aware that additional studies of its efficacy are needed.

2. Before taking PC SPES, undergo combination hormone therapy on a limited basis to reduce the PSA to below 4.0 ng/ml. Then discontinue CHT, and take three capsules of PC SPES along with an aspirin a day.

3. Prior to starting on PC SPES, get a baseline image of your disease so you can monitor the course of your recovery.

4. A medical doctor should oversee your treatment.

5. The first patient to undergo PC SPES for treating prostate cancer has taken these herbs for five years and has been off of this therapy for two more years without a recurrence of this disease. This may occur with you as well.

6. If and when your PSA goes to an undetectable level, an image study indicates no evidence of cancer, take a 5-region biopsy and stain the tissues, and observe each tissue under a microscope to see if cell death has occurred.

Chapter 7

THE BEST RADIATION TREATMENT FOR PROSTATE CANCER

prostRcision

If you learned that you could receive a radiation treatment for prostate cancer that is just as effective as or better than surgery, would you opt for it? You probably would say yes. Well, a treatment called *prostRcision* (PROS-tur-ci-shun) seems to achieve cure rates as good as, and in some cases better than, radical prostatectomy.

ProstRcision means excision of the prostate with radiation. ProstRcision's overall 10-year success rate of 72 percent is comparable to the eminent Dr. Patrick Walsh's 10-year success rate of 68 percent after radical prostatectomy, but the side effects of prostRcision are fewer. The 72 percent cancer-free rate of prostRcision patients includes all men regardless of their pretreatment PSA level (up to 188 ng/ml); it also includes men implanted by both the old open (retropubic) implant technique and the new ultrasound-guided transperineal implant. Men treated with prostRcision with the new transperineal method have significantly better cure rates. In addition, other factors indicate that prostRcision may indeed be better than surgery. Dr. Walsh carefully selects his patients. On the other hand, Dr. Frank Critz of the Radiotherapy Clinics of Georgia in Atlanta treats all patients who come to him regardless of their PSA before treatment, Gleason score, or stage.

ProstRcision, an integration of iodine seed implant and external beam radiation, is tailored to each individual patient through the use of a computerized database with more than 1.5 million entries. The database is invaluable because it allows the doctors at Radiotherapy Clinics of Georgia to plan and adjust the treatment for each individual patient. Dr. Critz performs an ultrasound-guided seed implant initially, and three weeks later, conformal beam radiation is delivered by a linear accelerator to intensify the radiation dose inside the prostate. In addition, the accelerator radiation treats cancer cells that may have gone through the wall (capsule) of the prostate because these cancer cells are not destroyed by seed implant alone. Critz places seeds in the seminal vesicles in case cancer cells have extended into this area. Some doctors say this dual dose of radiation is overkill. Well, we would rather have an overkill of these dangerous cells than an underkill. Remember, cancer cells that penetrate the prostate capsule are the ones that typically spread to lymph nodes and bones and eventually cause death.

Failed radical prostatectomy patients also go to Dr. Critz for treatment. Critz is the only radiation oncologist in the United States to perfect a treatment for patients who have failed surgery. Some radiologists have doubts about the effectiveness of his protocol, primarily because they do not know how to perform prostRcision and do not have the computerized prostRcision database.

We believe prostRcision is the "best" technique for radiating prostate cancer based on (1) our analysis of Dr. Critz's peer-reviewed medical research papers published in major medical journals and (2) a visit to Dr. Critz's facility. The prestigious medical journal, the *Cancer Journal From Scientific American*, published Dr. Critz's cancer-free rates in the November/December 1998 issue. Any man diagnosed with prostate cancer should read this paper thoroughly. It can be obtained from the medical library of most hospitals, from the *Cancer Journal from Scientific American*, or from Dr. Critz's office.

Dr. Critz's group analyzed 1,020 men treated between January 1984 and December 1996 who had stage T1T2N0 prostate cancer. All men initially underwent a radioactive Iodine-125 seed implant followed 3 weeks later by 6 to 7 weeks of external beam radiation given with a linear accelerator. Of the 1,020 men, 363 had the old retropubic implant technique and the remainder had the ultrasound guided implant. Almost all of these men had a seminal-vesicle implant. The median PSA was 7.5 ng/ml before pretreatment. None of these men received hormones. The overall 10-year cancer-free survival rate is 72 percent, after which a plateau is reached, indicating cure.

When the 1,020 men are divided according to whether they had the old implant technique or the newer ultrasound-guided implant followed by conformal beam radiation, even better results are shown. At 5 years after treatment, 92 percent of men treated with prostRcision by the ultrasound implant technique were free of cancer compared with 73 percent treated with the retropubic implant. This observation is important: it means that the overall cure rates of men treated with prostRcision by Dr. Critz are going to be significantly better than 72 percent when men treated with the ultrasound implant reach 10-year follow-up. Therefore, we expect the 10-year cure rates in Dr. Critz's study to greatly improve in the next few years. Already the 72 percent cure rate is at least as good as that achieved with surgery.

Equally remarkable about Dr. Critz's study in the *Cancer Journal from Scientific American* is that, unlike any other radiation study previously published, he rigorously analyzed his cure rates. Dr. Critz's group considered men to be cancer-free only if they achieved and maintained a PSA nadir level of 0.5 ng/ml or less after treatment. We believe that using this definition is the only way to accurately measure how well prostate cancer is being cured by radiation. No other radiation oncology group in the United States uses this definition. Other doctors believe it is too strict, and they are afraid that it will lower their cure-rate claims.

However, Dr. Critz's group no longer uses a PSA of 0.5 ng/ml to calculate cure after radiotherapy. They now use 0.2 ng/ml. In a lecture at the 1999 American Urological Association (AUA) meeting in Dallas, Texas, Dr. Critz documented that, with rare exceptions, only men who achieve a PSA nadir of 0.2 ng/ml or less have a chance of being cured of prostate cancer with radiation. Following prostRcision with the ultrasound method, 97 percent of cancer-free men followed for 5 years achieved a PSA nadir of 0.2 or lower. Furthermore, Dr. Critz, using both retropubic and ultrasound implant methods, showed that 92 percent of men who achieve a PSA nadir of 0.2 ng/ml or less are cancer-free 10 years after radiation treatment compared with only 41 percent who achieve a nadir of 0.3 to 1.0 ng/ml. No one is cured if their nadir exceeds 1.0. These findings apparently apply to all methods of radiation—and especially to any seed-implantation technique. These findings are important to know because there is increasing evidence that many radiation techniques used today are not very effective in curing prostate cancer.

Consider an article by Harvard researchers published in the *Journal of the American Medical Association*. In this article, the cancer-free rates of men with prostate cancer treated by radical prostatectomy, external beam radiation, or transperineal seed implant alone were analyzed. The researchers maintain that prostate removal is probably the best choice for men with prostate cancer. The investigation found that transperineal ultrasound-guided seed implantation by itself was much less effective than surgery or external beam radiation. When the researchers compared surgery, external beam radiation, and seed implant alone in 1,872 men, they found that those who had surgery or external beam radiation were three times more likely to be cancer-free after 5 years than were men who had only seed implantation. The article indicated that the ineffectiveness of seed implant could be due to the fact that a few cancer cells may survive after a full course of treatment. The cancer-free rates for both external beam and seed implant would have been a lot worse if cancer freedom had been defined by a PSA nadir of 0.2 ng/ml or less, as Dr. Critz has suggested. On the other hand, we believe the results in this study would have been much different if the men had been treated by prostRcision.

A Brief History of prostRcision

Dr. Critz's group began prostate seed implantation in 1977 at the Radiotherapy Clinics of Georgia. At first, they performed seed implants alone, but soon realized that seed implants by themselves are an ineffective treatment for prostate cancer. In 1979, they began a pilot study of radioactive I–125 seed implantation followed by external beam radiation.

Also in the late 1970s and early 1980s, a research group from Missouri and another from Copenhagen tried iodine implants (using both the retropubic and transperineal methods) followed by external beam radiation. Both the Missouri and Copenhagen subjects had disastrous bowel and bladder complications. The groups stopped their research, and their high complication rates were published in medical journals. Over the years, doctors read these reports and concluded this procedure didn't work. As a result, no other group ever tried this treatment.

In contrast, Dr. Critz's group, in pilot study, found this procedure could be done using a different technical combination method. In January 1984, they began a formal study of prostRcision that has continued to the present. They kept careful records of different radiation doses and techniques, how well patients were cured, and side effects of treatment. They entered all this information, accumulated since the early 1980s, into the prostRcision database. Using this database, the prostRcision technique was continually refined. They did not publish their first research paper until 1995 when they had over 10 years of follow-up. They wanted to first make certain that prostRcision cured prostate cancer.

As a result, the doctors at the Radiotherapy Clinics of Georgia are the only group to ever perfect prostRcision and they are the only group in the United States who use it. Since 1984, a total of 3,000 patients have been treated with prostRcision at the Radiotherapy Clinics of Georgia. This group has not only the oldest but also the largest single institution study on radiation for prostate cancer in the United States. They have been continuously performing seed implantation longer than any group in the United States.

Cancer Staging: An Educated Guess

In order to understand prostRcision, you first need to know how prostate cancer works. Prostate cancer goes through three phases:

Initially, one or more normal cells within the prostate gland transform into cancer cells. These cancer cells then multiply inside the prostate, but remain enclosed by a thin wall around the prostate called the *capsule*.

In the second phase, cancer cells inside the prostate penetrate the capsule of the prostate and spread into the surrounding organs: the rectum, bladder, sphincter muscles, sex nerves, and seminal vesicles. (These cancer cells, called *microscopic capsule-penetration cancer cells*, can be discovered with a microscope only after radical prostatectomy.)

Microscopic capsule-penetration cancer cells then spread (i.e., metastasize) through the lymphatic system and blood vessels into lymph nodes, bone, and throughout a man's body.

In order to treat a man diagnosed with prostate cancer, the doctor must first find out where the cancer cells are located. Obviously, the prostate biopsy indicates that there are cancer cells inside the prostate. The big question is whether the cancer cells have penetrated the capsule and whether they have metastasized.

Manual examination of the prostate (the DRE), and at times CT scans, MRI scans, and ProstaScint scans are performed to try to determine whether the cancer has penetrated the prostate capsule.

To check for metastasis, a bone scan may be performed. Occasionally, pelvic lymph nodes may be removed by a surgical procedure called a *pelvic node dissection*. However, most men diagnosed today do not need these procedures because the chance of finding metastases is so slim.

To indicate where prostate cancer cells are located, a staging system was devised. When men are believed to have cancer only in the prostate gland, we classify them as having *stage T1* or *stage T2* prostate cancer. If it is known before treatment that cancer cells have penetrated the capsule, men are classified *stage T3*. Today, almost all men are classified stage T1 or T2. Few men are classified before treatment as stage T3.

However, the staging system is highly inaccurate. When a patient is classified with stage T1 or T2 prostate cancer, this means that the doctor is just guessing that the cancer has not penetrated the capsule. Unfortunately, doctors often guess wrong. In fact, they guess wrong 50 percent of the time. Even with the digital exam, CAT scans, MRI scans, and prostaScint scans, there is absolutely no way to know or sure whether prostate cancer cells have spread beyond the capsule and spread into the adjacent bladder, rectum, or sphincter muscles.

How inaccurately doctors determine staging before treatment can be seen from the Partin Tables. The Partin Tables were compiled from patients who had a radical prostatectomy for what was thought to be stage T1 and T2 cancer. After surgery, the entire prostate specimen was carefully examined under a microscope by pathologists. They found that at least 50 percent of the men actually had cancer that had penetrated the prostate capsule and spread into the surrounding organs. These men were then classified as stage T3.

However, even the Partin Tables are not perfect. Up to 15 to 20 percent of men with cancer cells determined microscopically to be only in the prostate (i.e., *organ-confined*) fail to be cured by radical prostatectomy. Thus these patients had capsule penetration that could not be found even with microscopic examination of the entire prostate. So even if we could examine the prostate under a microscope *before* treatment, we would be guessing wrong about capsule penetration up to 20 percent of the time.

Although the Partin Tables are not perfect, they are still the best way to determine the chance of capsule penetration. The chance that cancer cells have penetrated the capsule and gone into the surrounding organs is related to the PSA level before treatment, as shown in Table 7-1.

Using this summary of the Partin Tables, you can see how often doctors guess incorrectly about where cancer cells are located. Even 25 percent of patients with what we think to be very early prostate cancer—those with a pre-treatment PSA level of 4.0 ng/ml or less—actually have cancer cells that have penetrated the prostate capsule. This information is important to any patient newly diagnosed

Table 7-1 PSA Level and Capsular Penetration

PSA of Men With Stage T1 and T2 before Prostatectomy (ng/ml)	Percent of Men After Surgery With Microscopic Capsule Penetration
4.0 or less	25%
4.1 to 10.0	50%
10.1 to 20.0	75%
More than 20.0	90%

with prostate cancer because cells will be missed and therefore not treated if doctors guess wrong about cancer-cell location. Undertreatment of prostate cancer is one of the worst things a doctor can do.

Principles of prostRcision:
I-125 Transperineal Seed Implant

ProstRcision eliminates the guesswork of clinical staging by accepting that half of men with stage T1 and T2 cancer actually are microscopic stage T3.

ProstRcision consists of an integration of two separate methods of irradiation: radioactive iodine seed implant followed by 3D conformal beam radiation. Both of these treatment methods undertreat prostate cancer when given alone; however, when integrated by the process of prostRcision, very high cure rates are achieved. The first part of prostRcision consists of a radioactive iodine seed implant. Radioactive iodine seeds are tiny pieces of metal that measure 4.5 mm long and 1 mm wide. These I-125 seeds have three important characteristics:

1. Each seed radiates only a very small area.

2. Seeds produce radiation for approximately one year.

3. The metal seeds are easily seen on x-rays.

Each radioactive iodine seed produces a tremendous amount of radiation to an area about the size of the tip of your small finger. Beyond this small area, the radiation drops off rapidly. By placing multiple seeds (an average of 90) throughout the prostate gland, a high dose of radiation is delivered within the prostate; however, the radiation dose drops sharply at the prostate capsule so that the adjacent bladder and rectum are not damaged.

On the other hand, prostate cancer cells that have penetrated the capsule will not be effectively treated. Therefore, since approximately 50 percent of men with stage T1 or T2 prostate cancer have microscopic capsule penetration, these men will be undertreated by ultrasound-guided seed implantation alone. (This observation applies to iodine seed implants, palladium seed implants, or any other radioactive seed implant).

The preceeding information corresponds to the rate of failure after ultrasound-guided transperineal seed implantation alone. Seed implants alone do not treat cancer cells that have penetrated the capsule, and many times cancer inside the prostate gland is also not cured. In a study of men with a Gleason score 6 or less by Dr. Haakon Ragde and Dr. John Blasko from Seattle, more than half were not cured after treatment with an ultrasound transperineal iodine implant alone (with cancer freedom calculated by a PSA nadir of 0.2 ng/ml). In a separate study from Florida, written by Dr. Jerrold Sharkey, again of highly selected men (those with a pretreatment PSA level between 4.0 and 10.0 ng/ml), 50 percent had a regrowth of cancer within 3 years of treatment with a palladium seed implant alone (with cancer freedom calculated by a PSA nadir 1.5 ng/ml).

Using either I-125 or palladium seed implant only, Dr. Nelson Stone observed a 24 percent failure rate only 2 years after implant (with cancer freedom calculated by PSA nadir of 1.0 ng/ml). These failure rates by Drs. Sharkey and Stone would have been a lot worse had they calculated cancer freedom using a PSA nadir of 0.2.

The failure rate of seed implant alone roughly corresponds to the percentage of men staged as T1 and T2 who actually have microscopic capsule penetration (stage T3).

Principles of prostRcision:
Precision Conformal Beam Radiaton

In order to compensate for the undertreatment of prostate cancer by ultrasound-guided seed implant alone, precision conformal beam radiation is given after the implant, which is the second part of prostRcision. Conformal beam radiation is given by a linear accelerator and is started three weeks after the implants. There are two fundamental reasons for follow up conformal beam radiation.

1. It intensifies the radiation dose inside the prostate.

2. It irradiates microscopic capsule-penetration cancer.

To understand this process, remember that radioactive iodine has a 2-month half-life, and therefore it produces irradiation for approximately one year. Since conformal beam radiation is started 3 weeks after the seed implant and is given for 6 to 7 weeks, both cancerous cells inside the prostate and normal prostate cells are irradiated simultaneously. This intensifies the radiation dose given to both normal and cancer cells. Radiation-dose intensification is needed inside the prostate because this is where prostate cancer started, this is where biopsies show cancer, and this is where the majority of cancer cells are located. In other words, the follow-up conformal beam radiation activates the radioactive iodine seeds.

Of equal importance, conformal beam radiation also treats cancer cells that have penetrated through the prostate capsule. Since only microscopic amounts of cancer cells extend through the capsule in men with (otherwise) stage T1 and T2 cancer, conformal beam radiation by itself can destroy these cancer cells. Therefore, prostRcision treats all known cancer cells inside the prostate and all microscopic cancer cells that have penetrated the capsule and spread into the rectum, bladder, sphincter muscles, and sex nerves.

Additionally, you should know that the prostate gland does not show up on X-rays. However, the metallic iodine seeds can easily be seen on an X-ray. The seeds are inserted throughout the prostate and seminal vesicles and outline these structures. Therefore, the iodine seeds are used as a target to deliver very precise conformal beam radiation.

Conformal beam radiation by itself fails to cure prostate cancer because of the limitations of the radiation dose since all radiation comes from the linear accelerator. The urethra, bladder, and rectum get the same dose of radiation that the cancer gets with conformal beam radiation only. As a result, it is usually not possible to give enough radiation to destroy the cancer without severely damaging the rectum and bladder, or urethra. In contrast, the dose of radiation can be tripled with prostRcision in the area of the cancer compared with conformal beam radiation because seeds are placed in the middle of the cancerous area noted by the sextant biopsy report.

The Concept of prostRcision:
Logical Integration

Using the computerized prostRcision database, prostRcision integrates two totally different forms of radiation that, by themselves, are ineffective treatments for stage T1 and T2 prostate cancer. When properly performed, prostRcision produces the highest radiation cure rate ever published. The principles of prostRcision are best summarized as:

1. Radiation dose is intensified inside the prostate where the majority of cancer cells are located.

2. Radiation of microscopic capsule-penetration cancer, is radiated for stage T3 cancer.

3. Precision conformal beam radiation allows for targeting the metal seeds.

4. The treatment is tailored to each individual patient using the computerized prostRcision database.

ProstRcision integrates transperineal iodine seed implant with conformal beam radiation using a highly logical and methodical process. In other words, prostRcision makes common sense.

Dr. Critz's group believes that doctors should accurately and realistically calculate cure rates for prostate cancer. Doctors should not be afraid to analyze their cure rates after radiotherapy by requiring that men achieve and maintain an undetectable PSA nadir. They should have enough courage to find out which radiation treatments are actually curing cancer. If some treatments are not very effective, patients should be told this. Accurate calculation of cure rates after any radiotherapy method is extremely important to any man with prostate cancer who is trying to decide on treatment. Remember, with rare exceptions, men with prostate cancer will get only one chance to be cured.

prostRcision Cure Rates

For men to be considered cured by prostRcision, they must achieve and maintain an undetectable PSA nadir of 0.2 ng/ml or less, the same definition of cure used by urologists after radical prostatectomy. Using this definition, the overall cure rate for men with stage T1 and T2 prostate cancer treated by prostRcision at Radiotherapy Clinics of Georgia is

66 percent at 10 years and also 15 years after treatment. This includes all men who were treated since 1984. None of these men were carefully selected for treatment, and none received hormones. The average PSA before treatment for all men was 12.2 ng/ml, with PSAs before treatment ranging up to 188 ng/ml. No one was turned away because of his Gleason score.

However the 66 percent overall cure rate includes men treated by the old, low-dose, obsolete open (retropubic) implant technique and men treated with the new high-dose ultrasound-guided transperineal implant technique. This is extremely important to understand because men treated by the old technique received half the amount of radiation as did men with the newer transperineal implant technique. The open implant method was stopped several years ago. Nonetheless, the 66 percent cure rate 10 years after prostRcision is just as good as the 68 percent achieved with radical prostatectomy at John Hopkins.

The 66 percent cure rate does not really reflect the cure rate at the Radiotherapy Clinics of Georgia. For several years, men with prostate cancer have been treated at the Radiotherapy Clinics with prostRcision using the new, high-dose ultrasound-guided transperineal implant method. Analyzing the cure rates of these men shows what prostRcision can really accomplish. The doctors expected a rise in cure rates using prostRcision with the transperineal implant technique, and this is exactly what they have seen. Five years after treatment with prostRcision using the ultrasound-guided transperineal implant technique, 90 percent of men are free of cancer (i.e., they have a PSA nadir of 0.2 ng/ml or lower). This cure rate is markedly improved over the 5-year cure rate with prostRcision using the old implant technique, which is 67 percent. Although 10-year cure rates are not available yet with prostRcision using the new transperineal implant technique, marked improvement is expected.

To be more specific, the cure rates calculated by a PSA nadir of 0.2 ng/ml with prostRcision using the ultrasound-guided implant technique at 5-year follow-up according to pretreatment PSA is given in Table 8.2. These are the highest cure rates ever seen for radiotherapy of prostate cancer.

Table 8-2. Cure Rates for ProstRcison at Various PSA Levels

Pretreatment PSA (ng/ml)	Cure Rate
4 or less	97%
4.0 to 10.0	92%
10.1 to 20.0	80%
More than 20.0	78%

African Americans and prostRcision

For reasons not fully understood, prostate cancer is often more advanced in African American men newly diagnosed with prostate cancer than it is in Caucasian men. African American men usually have a higher PSA before treatment than white men. Thus, in African-American men, prostate cancer is more likely to have penetrated the prostate capsule and perhaps spread to other places. In medical studies of cure rates after radical prostatectomy as well as after seed implantation alone, white men have a significantly better cure rate than do black men.

Just like at other institutions, newly diagnosed African American men with prostate cancer seen at the Radiotherapy Clinics of Georgia usually have a significantly higher PSA than newly diagnosed Caucasian men. This indicates more extensive disease, especially a greater chance of capsule penetration. However, in contrast to all other institutions, when treated with prostRcision, African American men have cure rates equal to those of white men.

Equality of cure rates is achieved because prostRcision treats both cancer cells inside the prostate as well as those microscopic cancer cells that have penetrated the prostate capsule. In other words, prostRcision compensates for the more advanced disease typically seen in black men.

It should be emphasized that a PSA nadir of 0.2 ng/ml or lower is used to calculate the cure rates for African American men. Except for radical prostatectomy reports, no other radiotherapy group has calculated cure rates for black men using a PSA nadir of 0.2 ng/ml. Therefore, using the identical undetectable PSA nadir goal for both black men and white men, the cure rates for both races are equal if men are treated with prostRcision. These research findings were presented at the May 1999 American Society of Clinical (ASCO) meeting in Atlanta.

Validation of the Principles of prostRcision

With prostRcision, the radiation dose is intensified inside the prostate where the majority of cancer cells are located, and microscopic penetration of cancer cells through the prostate capsule (which occurs in half of men with stage T1 and T2) is treated by the conformal beam. Thus, all known cancer, as well as highly probable areas of cancer, are treated. Prostate cancer is not undertreated because of doctors guessing wrong. The dose intensification also destroys all, or virtually all, normal prostate cells, which prevents development of new cancer.

These observations are validated by the fact that 90 percent of men treated with prostRcision using the ultrasound-guided transperineal implant technique have achieved and maintained a PSA nadir of 0.2 ng/ml or lower 5 years after treatment. Virtually all of the 10 percent of patients who were not cured by prostRcision failed because of metastases to bone that could not be found when they were treated but which showed up within 5 years of treatment.

In contrast, 50 percent of men, even though highly selected for very early cancer, when treated with ultrasound-guided transperineal seed implant alone (iodine or palladium) are not cured. The primary reason seed implants alone fail is that microscopic cancer cells have penetrated the prostate capsule and are not treated.

No report has been published analyzing the conformal beam radiation cure rate using an undetectable PSA nadir. However, one report was published analyzing cure rates after external beam radiation using a PSA nadir of 0.5 ng/ml. It showed only a 10 percent cure rate at 10 years after external beam radiation. Prostate biopsies of these men after treatment usually show persistent cancer cells inside the prostate because of the limitation of radiation dose with external beam technique, due to the urethra in the center of the prostate.

Hormones With Radiotherapy

Hormones (e.g., Lupron, Zoladex, Casodex, Eulixin, PC SPES) are not given with prostRcision. In fact, if men wish to be treated with prostRcision, they are asked not to go on hormones. If men have been taking hormones prior to contacting the Radiotherapy Clinics, they are asked to stop them. Dr. Critz's group has four solid reasons for not using hormones with prostRcision:

1. Doctors recommend hormones with radiotherapy because of two recently published studies combined with conventional external beam radiation. One study was done in Europe, and the other study was done by the Radiation Therapy Oncology Group in the United States. Both studies are seriously flawed because the radiotherapy technique used was the old-fashioned, conventional, external beam radiation. This is an obsolete treatment and the cure rate is only 10 per-

cent. ProstRcision is totally different: it cures prostate cancer, and the cure rate is 90 percent.

2. If hormones are given with a treatment method that cures prostate cancer, no benefit is seen. Radical prostatectomy can cure prostate cancer. However, published medical reports of hormones given with radical prostatectomy show no improvement in cure rates when compared with radical prostatectomy alone.

3. A number of men who received hormones prior to being seen at the Radiotherapy Clinics were treated with prostRcision after hormones were stopped. Cure-rates have been calculated for this group and compared with men who received prostRcision only. As with the surgical series, there is no difference in cure rates. Hormones did not help prostRcision.

4. Hormones cause a lot of complications. First, hormones ruin the results of the PSA test, artificially causing the PSA to fall to low levels. Thus, use of the PSA nadir test is ruined. Remember, the PSA nadir test is the single most important test result after any treatment for prostate cancer. In addition, hormones cause impotence and hot flashes, and if given long enough, can cause muscle weakening and thinning of the bones, making them break easier. Hormones can also shrink the prostate too much so that there is no place in which to put the seeds without jamming them right up against the urethra and rectum. This only causes more complications. For these reasons, Dr. Critz's group do not use hormones.

Some doctors give hormones when the radiation method they are using is not very effective. Doctors also give hormones when they have been undertrained and do not know what to do.

Contacting the Radiotherapy Clinics of Georgia

You can contact Radiotherapy Clinics of Georgia (RCOG) in order to get an information packet about prostRcision by visiting their website at or by phoning 404-320-1550 or 1-800-952-7687.

Records Needed for Pretreatment Evaluation

If you decide to ask the Radiotherapy Clinics to evaluate your case they will ask you to send certain records. These include all PSA reports, biopsy reports, pathology slides, scan reports, and any reports of other significant medical conditions. In addition, they will ask you to undergo a pelvic CT scan and send the actual images. This scan is important as it is used to measure the prostate size and shape and also to verify that the pelvic bones do not block access to the prostate.

To properly diagnose your condition, you will be asked to complete three comprehensive questionnaires:

1. *American Urological Association (AUA) Symptom Index*
   This instrument is used to evaluate urinary obstructive symptoms, such as BPH might cause.

2. *RCOG Comprehensive Assessment of Patient Symptoms (RCOG CAPS)*
   These 21-questions explore urinary irritative symptoms, quality of sex function, and rectal symptoms. Medication usage and prior pelvic surgical procedures are included as well.

3. *A questionnaire on sexual function.*
   Together, these questionnaires provide a comprehensive pretreatment profile of your urinary, sex-

ual, and rectal function. All information is entered into the RCOG computerized prostRcision database. Your profile can then be compared with the profiles of all the men previously treated at RCOG. In this way, the method of prostRcision can be tailored to your exact needs, and your possible reactions can be anticipated. The same questionnaires are used to follow your progress both during treatment and after it is completed. This comprehensive evaluation system forms the cornerstone of continuous improvement for patients treated at RCOG.

Weekly Prostate Cancer Conference

Once your materials are received at RCOG, a physician will evaluate them. The review will evaluate how the cancer was detected, PSA reports, pathology and X-ray reports, and the CT scan. It will also review the questionnaires. Your case will then be presented at the weekly Prostate Cancer Conference attended by all the doctors at RCOG. All treatment options will be considered not just prostRcision.

The particulars of your case will be compared with information from the RCOG computerized prostRcision database. Your PSA, Gleason score, stage, and questionnaire finds will be compared with those of thousands of men previously treated at RCOG with prostRcision. By doing this, the doctors at RCOG can predict what your cure rate will be and whether you will have any change in urinary, rectal, and sexual function. For example, a change in how often you need to get up at night to urinate can be predicted both during and after treatment.

Please note that all men are considered for prostRcision, regardless of the extent of their prostate cancer. Dr. Critz's group believes that all men deserve a chance to be cured, regardless of how bad their cancer is. The only exclusion is a patient whose prostate cancer has spread to the bones.

Furthermore, men are considered for prostRcision regardless of prostate size. Some doctors have said that implants cannot be done if the prostate size is above 50 or 60 cc. This is not correct. Because of their experience with several thousand patients, the RCOG doctors have implanted prostates larger than 160 cc.

On rare occasions, no more than 1 percent of the time, hormones have been given before the implant to shrink a massively enlarged prostate because or to treat severe BPH urinary obstructive symptoms. This differs from giving hormones to treat cancer, which is not done. The conference will make the decision on hormone treatment.

Contact by Doctor

After your case has been presented at the Prostate Cancer Conference, a doctor will contact you to discuss the indications, risks, and benefits of prostRcision as well as alternative treatments such as radical prostatectomy, watchful waiting, and if cancer has metastasized hormonal therapy.

This is not a formal consultation, and you are not charged for this call.

Visiting Atlanta

Before making a decision regarding treatment of your prostate cancer, you can visit Atlanta for a consultation. You will be seen by one of the physicians on the staff of the Radiotherapy Clinics. You may then return home and decide how you wish to be treated. On the other hand, if you have already decided to be treated at Radiotherapy Clinics, an initial trip is not necessary.

If prostRcision is the agreed-upon treatment, you may expect the seed-implant portion of prostRcision to be scheduled within 3 to 6 weeks. The staff will provide a listing of accommodations for the stay in Atlanta, and while you must make your own arrangements for lodging, a patient facilitator will provide helpful information.

Preparing for Treatment

Once you arrive in Atlanta, you will have a consultation with a radiation oncologist from RCOG, a urologist, and an anesthesiologist. The doctors at Radiotherapy Clinics of Georgia work with 40 urologists in Atlanta. It should be emphasized that you will be treated by a team approach. Both the urologist and radiation oncologist will again review with you the rationale and techniques of prostRcision and also the rationale and techniques of radical prostatectomy to make certain that you have made the choice that is best for you.

Seed Implant

Once your films and records have been reviewed in the weekly RCOG Prostate Cancer Conference and you have been accepted for treatment, the prostate implant is planned. While it may seem that most patients are similar, they are quite different in very important ways. For each patient, prostate gland size and shape vary as does the location of the urethra, and perhaps the relationship of the prostate to the rectum and bladder. The size and shape of the prostate and the extent of the cancer determine the total activity, number of seeds, and individual seed strength. All of these factors for each patient are related to the RCOG computerized database of all other men previously treated with prostRcision. Using all of this information, the doctors at RCOG then calculate how many seeds to order and where to place them in the prostate. Additionally, a computerized dosimetry plan is performed, outlining seed position for all seeds. Thus, two separate plans are made and are checked one against the other. However, each plan is only a rough guide to seed placement.

It is not until the patient is taken to the operating room and needles are inserted into the prostate that the final adjustments can be made. Urethral and rectal positioning, how the gland moves, and changes in response to the placement of the needles will affect the radiation oncologist's determination of the final seed distribution. The prostate gland is very mobile. It is also like an accordion, and it will stretch and contract and move. During the implant, doctors have to constantly adjust for all of these factors. Otherwise, seeds would be placed in the wrong location—either too far from the cancer or too close to the rectum, bladder, or urethra—and they will burn a hole in these normal organs. Finally, seed placement must allow for the follow-up conformal beam radiation. In all, a prostate seed implant is a very complex procedure and should be performed only by highly trained doctors.

A lot of doctors doing implants today do not understand all of this. These are the doctors who take a 2-day course in implants and think a computer plan can show them how to do them. These doctors use preloaded seeds and do not know about prostate gland motion or stretching. As a result, their seed implants do not cover the prostate. They do not know that extensive training is needed, constant use of the computerized prostRcision database.

Patients should stop all anticoagulation (blood-thinning) medicine, including aspirin and Coumadin, at least one week before the scheduled implant. Be sure to tell the doctors if you are taking such medicine. The day before your implant, you will be asked to drink some liquids and/or take an enema. Also, on the day before the procedure, drink only clear liquids after noon and then nothing by mouth past midnight. Do not eat or drink anything on the morning of the procedure.

Typical Implant Procedure

❏ 6:00 a.m.   Arrive at the hospital, and check into the outpatient surgery department.

❏ 6:30 a.m.   Change into a gown, and go to the waiting area. An IV is started, and the chart is checked to ensure that the consent for treatment is signed and the history and lab work are in order.

❏ 7:15 a.m.   Go to the operating room. Monitoring equipment is set up.

❏ 7:30 a.m.   Anesthesia, either general (preferred) or spinal (if medically necessary or if patient prefers) is started.

❏ 7:40 a.m.   The legs are placed in stirrups. The perineum, the area between the scrotum (bag) and the anus, is shaved to prevent contamination from hair. You are catheterized, and the pubic area is washed with an antibiotic solution. Drapes are then placed to maintain sterility, and the doctors begin their work.

❏ 7:50 a.m.   The radiation oncologist places the ultrasound probe into the rectum and fixes it into a special cradle. This allows the prostate to be precisely aligned with the implant grid. The rectum and urethra are identified and the location is marked. The location of the cancer is noted. The intraoperative findings are used to make changes in the pretreatment plans.

❏ 8:00 a.m.   Once all has been checked, the implant procedure begins. The doctors use a biplane ultrasound probe with multifrequency capability. Using the two preplans together with the intraoperative findings, the radiation oncologist and urologist jointly consult about placement of the needles, which are inserted from the bottom of the prostate (the apex) all the way to the top (the base) by the urologist. The needles are hollow and are 8 inches long. When the needles enter the prostate, they are seen on the ultrasound machine's screen and can be precisely positioned. Care is taken to encompass the entire prostate. The prostate is monitored for displacement, rotation, lift, tilt, and stretching while the needles are inserted, with adjustments again made relative to the preplan. If bone is hit, further adjustments are made. Doctors must have extensive training and experience to do this correctly.

❑ 8:10a.m.   After placement of the needles, the radiation oncologist performs a final adjustment to ensure that all areas of the gland are well covered. Then the actual insertion of seeds is begun. This is the most important and most difficult part of the entire procedure. If seeds are placed too far from the cancer, the patients will not be cured. If seeds are placed too close to normal organs, radiation will burn a hole in them. There is no room for error. Intensive training of the radiation oncologist in the precise placement of seeds is critical.

A device called a *seed gun*, is attached in sequence to each needle. Then the radiation oncologist begins injecting seeds. As the needles are slowly withdrawn, from two to seven seeds per needle are precisely injected in their appropriate locations. Some seeds will be placed close together in the area of cancer; other seeds will be placed further apart. This determination is made in the operating room.

Preloaded seeds in vicryl strands, such as Rapid Strand, are never used at RCOG because adjustments in seed location cannot be made. On average, 90 seeds are injected throughout the prostate. The seminal vesicles are also implanted to provide radiation to this critical region. The seeds in the seminal vesicles also serve as a target for subsequent boost treatment, if necessary.

❏ 8:25 a.m. After all the seeds have been inserted, the probe is withdrawn from the rectum. The urologist then performs a cystoscopy, inserting a small telescope into the bladder, to examine the bladder. The cystoscope is withdrawn, and a catheter is reinserted into the bladder.

The patient then goes to the recovery room, then to the outpatient area, and then home, or to his room, if he is spending the night in the hospital. On the day after surgery, postimplant CT scan is obtained. The catheter is removed, after evaluation of urinary flow, the patient returns home. Three weeks after the implant, precision conformal beam radiation is begun.

Precision Conformal Beam Radiation

ProstRcision is a complex process that involves great precision with both the seed implant and follow-up conformal beam radiation. Precision conformal beam radiation is given by a 24-MeV linear accelerator. These machines require precise alignment to the seeds coupled with the design of customized, individual blocking devices by the doctors to block out unnecessary radiation to the bladder, rectum, and sex nerves.

This process of precision alignment of the treatment set-up is called *simulation*. Simulation is performed on a Ximatron CX simulator and a dedicated CT scan simulator. Using laser beams, with the patient lying on the simulator machine, the prostate is precisely lined up using the seeds as a target. X-rays are made to confirm alignment. This process takes about 45 minutes. Small dots are drawn on the hips and belly to ensure proper alignment each time treatment is given. Computerized dosimetry plans are performed and approved, and then the first accelerator treatment is ready to be given.

You will be asked to lie down on the table of the linear accelerator. Again, using laser beams, the accelerator is aligned to the marks on your hips previously performed with simulation. An X-ray is taken to see that the seeds are aligned with the marks on your hips. The custom made blocks are then inserted into the accelerator, verification X-rays are made, and the actual radiation treatment is given. All you will hear is a buzzing or clicking sound.

Quality Control During Treatment

The quality of treatment delivery is rigidly and continuously monitored throughout conformal beam radiation by careful monitoring of patients. This is done in two ways.

1. When the block treatment is being given with the linear accelerator, X-rays are made with the linear accelerator machine at each day's treatment. These X-rays help ensure that the treatment machine will line up precisely on the prostate gland throughout your treatment. This is needed because the prostate moves.

   Without seeds outlining the prostate, doctors using ordinary conformal beam radiation treat a larger area in case the prostate gland moves. As a result, they often miss the cancer. All this does is unnecessarily irradiate the adjacent rectum and bladder and cause complications. Unlike all other radiotherapy facilities in the United States, at

Radiotherapy Clinics of Georgia, only the necessary area is irradiated.

2. The 21-question CAPS questionnaire is used to provide the second method of quality control. Each Monday, men answer the questionnaire before being treated. The questionnaire evaluates urinary, rectal, and sexual health. All of the previously treated men's answers have been entered into the RCOG prostRcision database. The weekly CAPS questionnaire is reviewed each Monday by a doctor with the patient, and adjustments are made, if needed, in how the conformal beam radiation is delivered. The answers of men currently under treatment are compared with the prostRcision database and serve as a guide in determining how the accelerator radiation is delivered, whether medication should be given, whether new blocks are needed, and whether machine angles should be changed. This quality control reduces the chance of complication from treatment.

Follow-Up

After treatment with prostRcision, men are followed for the rest of their lives by the Radiotherapy Clinics. Men who live in Atlanta or close to Atlanta are seen at the clinic for follow-up and men who live long distances and thus are not able to return to Atlanta are followed by telephone or mail.

All follow-up visits are dated from the month that the seed implant was done after finishing conformal beam radiation. The first follow-up visit called the 3-month follow-up, occurs approximately 2 weeks after the end of conformal beam radiation. Another follow-up visit is conducted 3 months later. All other follow-ups are then conducted at a6-month intervals.

At each follow-up visit, whether performed at the Radiotherapy Clinics or by phone or mail, a PSA is obtained and the AUA index, the CAPS, and sex-function questionnaires are filled out.

All the PSA data and questionnaire information at each follow-up are entered into the prostRcision database. By obtaining the questionnaires at the same follow-up intervals, a man's PSA and questionnaire answers can be compared with those of all of the men who have been previously treated at RCOG. This is extremely important because the doctors can determine what symptoms might be expected, what symptoms might not be expected, what medications to use, etc. Symptoms change with time. For example, the frequency of getting up at night to urinate will be different between the 6- and 12-month follow-up.

Medication That Interferes With the PSA Test

It is important that men who undergo prostRcision not take any medicine or supplement that will interfere with the PSA test. Remember, the PSA test after treatment is the best way to measure the destruction and death of the prostate cancer.

A number of drugs and supplements may artificially lower the PSA level. These drugs should be avoided. They include saw palmetto, Proscar, Propecia, and any drug containing hormones or estrogen.

Side Effects of prostRcision

Urinary problems are the most common side effects of prostRcision. Believe it or not, they are not due to radiation. Almost all urinary problems are due to trauma to the prostate caused by insertion of the 8-inch-long needles through which the seeds are injected. Typically 20 to 25 needles are inserted from the bottom of the prostate all the way to the top. The needles cause swelling of the prostate, which in turn compresses, or squeezes, the urethra, which runs through the middle of the prostate. As a result, men develop a weak, slow stream, have difficulty starting urination, have a greater urge to urinate, and have to urinate more frequently. Additionally, some men have discomfort when starting to urinate.

These symptoms typically start on the day following the implant, within hours after the catheter is removed. This occurs prior to conformal beam radiation and before hardly any radiation from the seeds has been implanted. The symptoms on average persist for approximately three months and then gradually subside as the prostate gland shrinks. Shrinkage takes about one year. The degree of urinary symptoms is usually related to the size of the prostate before treatment and preexisting urinary symptoms. Men with normal-size prostates with hardly any urinary symptoms before treatment usually experience very few urinary symptoms after prostRcision. On the other hand, men with enlarged prostates and/or severe urinary obstructive symptoms to begin with, are those who typically get the worst urinary symptoms.

However, the amount of swelling of the prostate varies greatly from man to man. Even some men with normal-size prostates with few urinary symptoms will still develop tremendous swelling of the prostate and will have considerable urinary symptoms after the seed implant. Swelling of the prostate occurs after any form of seed implantation whether as part of prostRcision or when seed implants are performed alone.

Additionally, about 4 percent of men have swelling of the prostate that may totally block the urethra. In this case, after the catheter is removed, it may need to be reinserted. If this happens, the average time to wear a catheter is 3 weeks.

A bruise is typically seen in a man's perineum after the implant. Also, it is common for men to see some blood in their urine for a few days to a few weeks. Again, this is from the needles being inserted. Men rarely have any pain after the implant. If they do, Tylenol is about all that is required. Men do not develop nausea or vomiting, or grow hair. Men can continue working at their usual jobs without interruption.

Sexual Activity

Sexual activity can be resumed within a day or so of the implant. A condom is not necessary. Men typically ejaculate bright red blood and then older blood for several weeks after the implant. Bleeding inside the prostate is caused by the needle insertion. Since semen is produced by normal prostate cells, the amount of semen gradually gets less and less. Occasionally, seeds are ejaculated. This will cause no harm to the man's partner and will be passed.

The ejaculatory ducts run inside the prostate and empty into the urethra in the middle of the prostate. Only on rare occasions do men have any significant pain with ejaculation. Except for occasional mild discomfort, patients usually notice no effect with ejaculation. Following prostRcision, 72 percent of who were sexually active before treatment maintained sexual function. However, about one-third of the patients have some erectile dysfunction. Viagra often helps them.

Rectal Complications

Rectal symptoms are most strongly influenced by a history of hemorrhoids. If you have a history of hemorrhoids, you may find an increase in symptoms during the 6 to 7 weeks of conformal beam irradiation. The most common symptoms requiring medication are a few drops of blood in the stool and discomfort with bowel movements. Few patients have required cortisone suppositories for rectal symptoms after treatment. Only one-tenth of one percent (0.1%) of men—one man—treated by prostRcision with the ultrasound implant method developed rectal damage requiring a colostomy.

Why prostRcision Is Performed
Only at the Radiotherapy Clinics

Other doctor groups have tried performing prostate iodine seed implant followed by linear accelerator radiation. As mentioned earlier, research groups from the University of Missouri and Copenhagen tried this approach in the 1970s and early 1980s but had disastrous rectal complications.

Doctors at the Radiotherapy Clinics have not had these complications because they are all highly trained in prostRcision, a rigid quality-control program is enforced, and doctors continuously use the prostRcision database to tailor treatment to each individual patient. This is also why Dr. Critz's group mandates that they give all radiation themselves. Years ago, they tried sending patients back home for the follow-up conformal radiation. However, they saw severe bladder and bowel complications in some patients who underwent radiation elsewhere. Staying in Atlanta for 6 weeks is a minor inconvenience compared to suffering severe and permanent damage to your rectum or bladder.

Activities After the Seed Implant

Following the seed implant, men can do almost anything they wish. However, they cannot sit on narrow, hard objects such as a bicycle seat for the first two months after the implant. Otherwise, there is no limitation on activity. Men may return to work, jogging, running, or any activity the day after the implant. There is no restriction during conformal beam radiation.

Does Radiation Cause Other Cancers?

There is no increased risk of secondary cancers as a result of radiation therapy to the prostate. However, men may still develop other cancers in the rectum and bladder as well as other sites unrelated to the prostRcision. Patients are encouraged to see their personal doctors for complete physicals each year.

Contact With Other People

The amount of radiation emitted by the Iodine-125 seeds is very low, and the body itself stops virtually all of the radiation. While a tiny amount of radiation does leave the body, it is so small that there are no restrictions on your daily activities and interaction with most people. However, precaution is advised when you are near small children and pregnant women. You can always give a child or pregnant woman a kiss and a hug, but if you are going to be in the same room for longer than 10 minutes or so per day, stay two or more feet away from them for the first two months after the implant. Do not let small children sit on your lap for the first two months.

Quality Control and Quality of Training of Doctors

RCOG has the highest standard for training of seed implantation of any institution in the United States. At RCOG, only doctors who have been highly trained are allowed to perform prostRcision, including both seed implantation and the follow-up conformal beam radiation. New doctors who join RCOG must observe at least six cases of both the seed implant and follow-up conformal beam radiation as performed by certified staff members. Then certified staff doctors directly supervise the new doctors while they perform at least 100 cases of seed implantation followed by conformal beam radiation. Throughout their training, new doctors are shown how to use the prostRcision database. Only doctors who undergo this rigid training and who have been certified to practice prost-Rcision are allowed to treat men with prostRcision. Doctors who have undergone only 2-day training courses are not acceptable at the Radiotherapy Clinics of Georgia.

Additionally, doctors are continuously monitored for quality control even after they have been certified to perform prostRcision at RCOG. This is done in two different ways. First, cure rates are continuously calculated for each individual doctor at RCOG and compared with those of all the other doctors at RCOG. Secondly, a weekly prostate Seed Implant Conference, including administration of conformal beam radiation, is held each week. All doctors at RCOG participate in this conference. All seed implants performed are reviewed as are plans for conformal beam radiation. Any doctor not performing prostRcision correctly is taken off the operation schedule and given further training.

Furthermore, as research is continuously being performed with the computerized database, continuous refinements are made in prostRcision and are implemented at the weekly Seed Implant Conference. Thus, prostRcision is always being refined, and all doctors at RCOG participate in a continuous learning process using data from the database. Doctors at RCOG undergo the highest standard of training in the United States and are continuously monitored to maintain this standard. Such quality is the backbone of prostRcision administered at the Radiotherapy Clinics.

It does not make any difference which doctor performs prostRcision at the Radiotherapy Clinics. All doctors perform prostRcision equally well, including the seed implant and the follow-up conformal beam radiation.

Why is quality training of doctors and continuous training so important? The answer is very simple. With few exceptions, men get only one chance to be cured of prostate cancer. If men with prostate cancer undergo radiotherapy, regardless of technique, and are not cured, they cannot be salvaged by radical prostatectomy or any other method except under rare circumstances and then only with extremely high complication rates.

In other words, if men with prostate cancer are not cured because they choose the wrong radiation technique, one that does not cure prostate cancer very well, or if they are treated by undertrained doctors who do not know what they are doing, these men can rarely be cured by a second treatment. If men fail to be cured with radiation, they are then sentenced to a lifetime of hormones. Hormones cannot cure prostate cancer but will typically suppress its growth for an average of four years, after which the cancer becomes resistant to hormones.

When men with prostate cancer choose any treatment program, especially radiotherapy, they should choose a treatment method with a proven peer-reviewed published cure rate that has been rigorously analyzed by 0.2 ng/ml. Additionally, they should be treated by doctors who know absolutely what they are doing and who maintain the highest standards of quality of training.

Many other doctors do not agree with Radiotherapy Clinics of Georgia regarding quality of treatment for prostate cancer. Obviously, some doctors will deny this, but look at what is done. Some doctors take a two-day seed-implant course that consists of no more than a few lectures, never do even one supervised seed implant, and either see someone else do one or two seed implants or just simply get a videotape of someone doing a seed implant. They pay $700 to $1,000 for this course and get a certificate that they can hang on their wall back home stating that they are now a seed-implant doctor.

Then with this quality of training and no computerized database, these doctors advertise that they offer seed implants for men with prostate cancer. They get a physicist to run a computer plan to show where the seeds should go.

The physicist—who has never been to medical school, knows nothing about prostate cancer, and has had no training in its treatment—tries to tell the doctors where to place the seeds. The doctors have no idea how to make adjustments in the operating room. It is like the blind leading the blind. All of this is going on today throughout the United States.

The undertraining of doctors may also explain why so many doctors recommend hormones with radiation. Patients can easily find out if they are being cured by getting PSA measurements after radiation and seeing what PSA nadir they achieve. However, when men are placed on hormones, the PSA test is temporarily ruined and the PSA nadir cannot be measured. Hormones are used to cover up the fact that patients are not cured because of undertraining of doctors.

Patients Who Cannot Afford prostRcision

For patients who do not have insurance and cannot afford to pay, RCOG provides treatment free of charge. Seed companies have been very good in providing seeds for such cases. Additionally, RCOG tries to find lodging in Atlanta at no charge. The only expense that might be needed would be transportation to and from Atlanta as well as meals in Atlanta.

Doctors Who are Critical of Radiotherapy Clinics of Georgia

Most doctors are highly complimentary of the research findings from Radiotherapy Clinics of Georgia and have the highest respect for Dr. Critz's group for challenging other radiotherapy doctors to have the same high-quality standards as at RCOG. However, some doctors say negative things about Dr. Critz's group. This is understandable for several reasons. Dr. Critz's group has strongly advocated strict and realistic standards for calculation of cure rates after radiotherapy originally using an endpoint PSA nadir of 0.5 ng/ml and now a PSA nadir of 0.2 ng/ml. All other doctors who have reported their cure rates after radiotherapy of prostate cancer object to this definition because it makes their cure rates worse. This challenge to other doctors to realistically analyze their cure rates has upset them.

Additionally, Dr. Critz's group advocates high standards for the training of doctors as well as continuous quality control. They have been critical of 2-day training courses after which doctors begin doing seed implants. They think this training is irresponsible and inadequate and have said so publicly. This also has angered many doctors. The doctors at Radiotherapy Clinics of Georgia also do not recommend giving hormones with prostRcision. Other doctors want to give hormones with radiation and get upset when the Georgia group challenges them.

Dr. Critz's group does not go along with the crowd; they challenge others to use high standards, and have produced the highest cure rates ever published. I personally visited Radiotherapy Clinics of Georgia and find them to back up everything they say with extensive research. Furthermore, all their research efforts have gone through a peer-review process before publication in major medical journals. If there was anything wrong with their research findings, their research papers would never have been published, nor would they be invited to make presentations at major medical meetings. So if you hear criticism of Radiotherapy Clinics of Georgia, ignore what you hear and make your own determination, better yet, call the author.

prostRcision as Salvage Treatment

Since many men treated for prostate cancer with other treatment methods (radical prostatectomy, cryosurgery, and other forms of radiation) are not cured, prostRcision has been used at RCOG to try to cure them.

In particular, prostRcision has been used in the treatment of men who are not cured by radical prostatectomy. It is very difficult to do a seed implant following a radical prostatectomy because the prostate is no longer present. Seeds are placed in the scar tissue where the prostate gland used to be, but this is a very highly specialized implant technique because the anatomy is changed following prostatectomy. The cure rates in this procedure are very promising.

Additionally, prostRcision has been used for cryosurgery failures, and failures after radiation. Again, because patients have already received a lot of radiation to the rectum and bladder, prostRcision under these circumstances is difficult to perform but can be performed successfully.

Summary

In summary, prostRcision is based upon a logical integration of radioactive iodine-seed implantation followed by conformal beam radiation. This produces radiation-dose intensification inside the prostate and treats microscopic extension of cancer cells through the prostate capsule, present in half of men with stage T1 and T2 disease. The principles of prostRcision are validated by the overall 90 percent cure rate at 5 years after treatment with the ultrasound implant technique.

An undetectable PSA nadir (0.2 ng/ml) after prostRcision is used to calculate cure rates, which is the identical definition for use in radical prostatectomy reports. Thus, prostRcision means a "radiation prostatectomy" but without removal of sex nerves or the muscles that control urination. ProstRcision means excision of the prostate with radiation.

The RCOG computerized database for prostRcision contains PSA levels and urinary, sexual, and rectal function data before, during, and after treatment for all men treated at RCOG. The database is an invaluable tool for the evaluation of new patients, conducting research and is the cornerstone to how to tailor treatment for each patient. The RCOG computerized database for prostate cancer is the largest database in the United States.

Quality control is the backbone to management of patients with prostRcision. Doctors are allowed to perform prostRcision only after extensive training. Men are monitored by the strictest degree of quality control with the emphasis not only on maximum cure rates but also on maintaining the highest quality of life.

If there is one word to sum up RCOG, it would be *precision*. Seed implants are precisely done for follow-up precision conformal radiation, given by doctors who are precisely trained. Cure rates are precisely calculated with an undetectable PSA nadir and urinary, rectal, and sexual function are precisely monitored with self-administered questionnaires.

Some doctors claim they specialize in treating prostate cancer. The doctors at Radiotherapy Clinics of Georgia specialize in curing prostate cancer. However there is a big difference.

Why We Selected This Treatment

We selected prostRcision as the best radiation treatment for prostate cancer for several reasons:

1. It has a 10-year statistical study of cure rates computed by an outside independent agency. Its cure rates are the highest ever published.

2. Men with advanced cancer are not rejected for treatment in order to increase cure rates.

3. It is a synergistic dose-intensifying treatment since the iodine implant is done before the conformal radiation.

4. All prostate cancer patients are treated as though they have microscopic capsule penetration (i.e., stage T3).

5. Doctors must be extensively trained; the requirement is at least 100 cases.

6. Patients report that the treatment environment is one of compassion.

7. It has the only radiation oncologists in the country who seed the seminal vesicles.

8. It's a viable option for failed radical prostatectomy patients.

9. The computerized prostRcision database is the oldest and most extensive in the United States.

How You Should Use This Information

It is suggested that you select prostRcision if you want the following:

1. To receive a radiation treatment that gets at least the identical success rate as surgery, but with fewer side effects.

2. To undergo a treatment that achieves the same results as a radical prostatectomy but does not affect the sex nerves or urinary function.

3. To possibly get a PSA nadir of 0.2 ng/ml or less.

4. To receive seeds in the seminal vesicles.

5. To be reseeded.

6. To get a seed implant after failing radiation.

7. To receive radiation treatment in a caring environment.

Chapter 8

THE BEST TREATMENT FOR MULTIPLE BONE SITES

Quadramet

Bone pain is the most common type of pain caused by prostate cancer. As a result, routine questions of each patient complaining of pain is extremely important because the symptoms are often insidious from the onset and may be attributed to a host of other bone diseases, such as old age, Paget's disease, and arthritis. Such a self-diagnosis may not be actually wrong, but it must not prevent doctors from accurate diagnosis of the pain being experienced by the patient and the professional assistance being offered. The description of the character of the pain varies with the individual patient. Different patients may use words which implies different or opposite characteristics, such as dull/red hot and aching/stabbing. An exaggeration of pain with movement or pressure is often common. Tenderness over a bone may indicate metastasis until proven otherwise. A normal radiological appearance cannot exclude a bone metastasis and an isotopic scan is usually much more sensitive. It is believed that a substance known as prostacyclins are liberated by most tumor deposits in bone causing both reabsorption of bone around the tumor and sensitivity of nerve endings to a painful stimuli. Bone metastasis therefore can cause when they are very small. When metastases enlarge, they cause destruction of the bone under stress and may lead to pathological fracture. Vertebral collapse may lead to nerve root pain.

Bone Pain Treatment Options

External beam radiation must be carefully considered for patients with bone pain. Solitary metastases in long bones respond well to single doses as to more prolonged causes. A half body radiation should be considered for widespread metastasis.

Hemibody Radiation

Spot radiation is certainly effective in palliating bone pain, however, it is not usual for multiple sites of bone metastasis to appear simultaneously or within a short period. If each site of bone pain is radiated on an individual level, the patient may be inconvenienced throughout the radiation period. Therefore, the hemibody radiation procedure seems like a logical alternative for patients who have multiple sites of bone pain. The field and dose of Gy should be delivered to one half of the body. If and when necessary, the second half of the body should not be treated simultaneously because the dose that can be applied safely to the whole body is much lower than that which can be delivered to half the body. Be mindful, that the dose for radiating the total body should not exceed 300 Gy in a single or fractionated dose because the effects of lethal toxicity. The upper half of the body field usually extends from above the scalp to the umbilicus and the lower half from the umbilicus to the ankles. Up to 30 minutes is required to do one half of the body. After 4 to 6 weeks, when the blood counts have returned to normal, the second half of the body can be treated. Complete pain relief has been reported in 24-70% of patients and partial pain relief in 24-71%. The average response time duration is 6 months but it does not stop additional use of localized therapy to the recurrence or new symptoms. Usually the timetable is commensurate to a majority of the patient's remaining life; therefore, the patient should be grateful that there is a period relatively free of pain because most of the patients will eventually become hormone resistant. Nevertheless, other forms of adjunctive systemic treatment may become progressively unpleasant.

Side effects of hemibody radiation are those usually occurring immediately after and up to 2 weeks post treatment. The symptoms may include nausea, vomiting, elevated temperature and pulse rate, hypertension, and less significant side effects of the hemibody radiation. After many years of experience, most radiotherapists agree that 600 cGy is sufficient for the upper half of the body and 800 cGy is sufficient for the lower half of the body. An alternate radiotherapy treatment which is useful in patients with widespread and painful bone metastasis is the intravenous use of strontium or quadramet.

This form of radiation therapy should be used to relieve not only specific symptoms, but for local and remote problems too. It is usually required when one hormonal or herbal treatment begins to fail but may sometimes have a place early in the management of a patient because hormonal and herbal treatment is much relative in its effect and an individual patient may be left with a local site of pain. Usually, relatively high dose of radiation must be used because the majority of prostate cancers are slow growing and require substantial radiation doses applied to provide significant regression. Sometimes, patients may live for several years, even though they may have significantly local metastasis. Therefore, radiation must be carefully applied in order to minimize the long-term effects of the radiation.

In fact the use of hemibody radiation and a radio-pharmaceutical usually results in higher response rate and less bone pain.

Radio-Pharmaceuticals for Bone Pain

Hemibody radiation is useful and effective in prostate cancer patients with diffused and rapidly recurrent pain, but it is also associated with a significant toxicity and is therefore difficult to repeat as a treatment. As a result, there exists a dire need for an effective and well tolerated systemic therapy that can go right to the site of need and can be repeated. A radio-pharmaceutical is a mode of action which lead to an efficient localization at the site of a bone metastases. It provides pain relief for a period of six months in 80 percent of patients with hormone resistant bone pain while causing a minimal of side effects through selective radiation of multiple sites simultaneously. It has also been used at an early stage in the disease process before the pain occurred in patients by citing it in a partial resolution bone on the bone scan. It is also a reasonable alternative to external beam radiation when it is not easily and readily available.

There a several forms of radionuclide treatments for metastatic bone pain sites such as strontium 89, Rhenium–186, and Samarium–153 (quadramet) but only two, strontium 89 and quadramet attack both lytic and blastic spread bone disease.

In 3 different clinical trials of strontium 89 and hormonal refractory patients, a decrease in bone pain occurred in 67–80% of the patients. Pain relief lasted from 3–6 months with 27% of the patients becoming pain-free. A temporary increase in pain or flare response was seen in 10% of patients. Pain response occurs about 7–20 days after strontium 89 was administered.

In a double-blind study centrally randomized 114 cancer patients with painful bone metastases received a single dose of quadramet. During the first 4 weeks after administration, patients assessed each day their intensity, daytime discomfort and ability to sleep. During the fourth week which was considered the primary efficacy time point of the study, there was a statistically-significant difference in pain relief between the two doses in favor of the 1.0 C1/Kg dose.

These doses should produce a tumor regression without injury to tissue. Single bone metastasis can usually be palliated by doses of 40 Gy in 4 weeks at the rate of 2 Gy per day.

One very important decision to make is everything should be done to prevent cord compression. As a result, areas of involvement in the vertebrae should be treated before structural damage threatens the integrity of the spinal cord. In order to halt the progression, the radiation dose must be relatively high, such as a dose of 40 to 50 Gy delivered at the rate of 2 Gy a day.

Spot Radiation

If you have pain in a concentrated area of the body, you should consider undergoing spot radiation. This form of radiation is similar to hemibody radiation treatment except that the radiation is directed to the specific site of the pain which may not necessarily target the cancer. The majority of patients (70 to 80 percent) who receive spot radiation indicate that they receive complete or partial pain relief. Spot radiation usually takes 10–20 days to provide pain relief and may last 4 to 15 months. The average decrease in platelet count post treatment is 24 to 50 percent.

Kinds of Cancer Damage to Bone Destruction

Prostate cancer cells spread in the body in two primary ways. The first way is through the lymphatic channels that drain the pelvic cavity. As a result, any cancerous cells in the pelvic lymph nodes is a definite marker for metastatic disease. The second way in which metastatic prostate cancer spreads is through the channel that drains blood from the pelvic area.

Metastases first infect the surrounding bone tissue by causing certain physiological changes to take place at the cellular level. As a result, chemicals secreted by the metastases stimulate unnatural bone growth and destruction. Usually, there is an imbalance toward abnormal new bone formation around the progression of the disease. This new bone tissue is overly dense and weaker than the normal bone. This abnormal growth is referred to as "blastic" bone change. It appears as whiter area on a plain film bone x-ray. The blastic outgrowth is in the confined marrow channel and the actual swelling mass of tumor will produce a pressure causing pain because the surface of the bone has nerve fibers.

The second type of metastatic change damage is destructive. Bone may become imbedded with holes, a process that undermines the integrity of essential bones of your legs, hips and spine. This form of metastatic bone destruction is referred to as "lytic" change. Lytic change does not appear on a bone scan like the blastic bone change. Therefore the plain film bone x-ray is an important diagnostic tool if lytic bone change is suspected.

What Patients are Claiming About Quadramet

"The pain that I would get in my back was just like a toothache. It would throb. If I was lying down, it would feel like it (the pain) was raising me up off the bed."

—L.R.

"Tried Darvoset (with no good results), Demerol (no good), time-released morphine (no more pain, but couldn't function from the tired side effect— listless)." "After I had the quadramet it was a lot easier to live with me because I wasn't constantly worrying about whether I was in pain or not. I now work part time and am feeling good."

—R.S.

"I'm just very grateful that they came out with the treatment when they did and that we were able to hear of it. The best thing that worked for me was the quadramet."

—L.R.

"We had been told that there wasn't anything else that the cancer doctors could do for the pain, and then like a Godsend, this quadramet was offered to us as a way of dealing with this problem. I can truthfully say that it has been a Godsend to us. My husband had not felt like visiting and with the quadramet he was able to do that again with some degree of comfort. We had heard about so many adverse effects about this problem that he had—the prostate cancer that has progressed to the bone— that we didn't know what to expect. This drug was so new to us that we didn't have anything to compare it with. We just knew what the doctor had told us. That it would hopefully reduce his pain and it did.

—J.S.

"I had quite a bit of pain before I had the injections. The pain came mostly at night. I had problems sleeping. After the injection, I was able to sleep again. I was very surprised that I was able to drive 800 miles to my son's house, which I wasn't sure that I would ever be able to make that drive again."

—M.S.

The Primary Goal for Treating Multiple Metastatic Bone Pain Sites

The only goal for treating metastatic bone pain sites is to improve survival and restore quality of like so that the patient experiencing the pain begins to feel good and survives in the process.

The following represents how strontium 89 compares to quadramet regarding the treatment of multiple bone pain sites:

1. *Relieved the patients with bone pain in the shortest time period.*

   Whereby strontium 89 relieves a greater number of patients with metastases bone pain compared to quadramet (67–80 vs. 70–75 respectively). Quadramet relieves patients with bone pain much sooner than strontium 89 (1 to 3 weeks vs. 3 to 6 months) with complete response in 25% of patients with strontium and about half of the patients on quadramet.

2. *The agent can be used to retreat the patient's bone pain in a short period of time.*

   Retreatment can be performed at intervals of not less than a mean duration of 90 days with strontium 89 and 56 days with Quadamet.

3. *A minimum of time should elapse before you begin the initial treatment of the patient and when he is to be retreated.*

A minimum of 7 days can elapse between treatment and retreatment with quadramet and 60–90 days with strontium 89.

4. *The patient should be able to undergo other drugs and treatment in the shortest period of time.*

   While patients undergoing strontium 89 other drugs cannot be administered or treatment before 30 days have elapsed, those on quadramet can within 7 days.

5. *The agent should have a short physical half life cycle.*

   The short physical half life of quadramet is 46.3 and the short physical life of strontium 89 is 50.5 days.

6. *White blood cell count should recover in a short period.*

   White blood cell count recurs with 4 to 6 weeks for strontium 89 and 3 to 5 weeks on quadramet.

7. *Platelet count should completely recover during a short period of time.*

   Platelet count recurs 12 weeks using strontium 89 and the lowest level of 40 to 50% of base within 3 to 5 weeks.

8. *Pain relief should last for the greatest duration.*

   Pain relief lasted for 3 to 6 weeks with strontium 89, 4 or more weeks with quadramet.

9. *The agent should reduce the need for other drugs.*

   Approximately half of the patients reduced opioid usage by the 4th week on quadramet. No figures were available for strontium 89.

10. *The patient experiencing the multiple metastatic bone pain should begin to feel good in the shortest time period.*

   Whereby strontium 89 relieves a *greater number* of patients with metastatic bone pain compared to quadramet (67–80 percent vs. 48–54 percent respectively). Quadramet relieves patients with bone pain much sooner than strontium 89—3 weeks vs. 3–6 months.

11. *The agent can be used to retreat the patient in a time period of 90 days—strontium/quadramet. A minimum of time should elapse before being retreating.*

   A minimum of 7 days relapsed before being retreated with quadramet while a minimum of 3 months must have elapsed for strontium 89.

Conclusion

A greater number of patients may be treated for bone pain with strontium 89; however in most critical cases quadramet appears to present an improvement over strontium 89 In Most Categories Cited In Analysis.

Why I Selected this Treatment for Multiple Metastases Bone Pain Sites

Any patient experiencing multiple metastases bone pain sites desire a medication that can be administered by a single injection, thus causing pain relief in the shortest period of time, able to attack both lytic and blastic bone structure, has a short physical half-life cycle, and the patient is able to undergo another drug or treatment in a short period of time. The quadramet appears to meet many of these criterion.

How You May Use This Information

If you have multiple metastases bone pain sites and desire to use radio-pharmaceuticals to relieve your pain, you may be able to improve the efficacy of quadramet by adding hemibody radiation to areas affected.

If another treatment is necessary, wait 7 days before retreatment.

Chapter 9

The Best Combination of Drugs for Prostate Cancer

Clinical Synergism

In the "first generation" of chemotherapy, single agents, such as nitrogen mustard, methotrexate, and cyclophosphamide were not effective. However, in the second and third generations, single drugs were combined in a complicated regimen, at high doses, in an attempt to overcome drug resistance. About thirty years ago, this use of such combination "cocktails" became a firm foundation for guiding principles of chemotherapy. Although combination chemotherapy is more effective than single-agent therapy in advanced prostate cancer, it does not usually result in increased survival for patients.

Other drugs are commonly added to agents to produce meaningful combination "cocktails." However, these "cocktails" must be approached with care and must be geared to the needs of individual patients. They have many complications. Chemotherapy can have a wide range of toxicity.

Some side effects are hair loss, mouth sores, nausea and vomiting. The drugs themselves may be a source of future problems. Not all effects of these drugs are immediately obvious. Most of these drugs are considered *cytotoxic*—that is they are poisonous, not just to cancer cells, but to healthy cells as well. Knowing all of the complications with chemotherapeutic drugs, the first and most important task of the doctor and the patient former, is to agree to a combination "cocktail"—one which is best suited to the need of the patient, that will offer the patient the highest response, give a comfortable quality of life and, if possible, extend survival.

Pertinent Terminology In Chemotherapy

The following terminology will help you gain a better understanding of chemotherapy.

Response Rate

A *response* is the shrinkage of tumors by 50 percent or more for at least one month. When doctors describe a treatment as having an excellent *response rate*, this may not necessarily correlate with an increase in overall survival. For many cancers, a response is not equal to better survival. However, at a meeting of the American Society for Clinical Oncology, many of the presenters indicated that "response rates" determine the effectiveness of chemotherapeutic drugs.

One fallacy of chemotherapy is that shrinkages or "response rates" have been shown to correlate with increased survival time. When a patient questions an oncologist about the chances of his survival, some doctors may answer, "The response rate is 73 percent," without explaining what a response rate is or how it correlates with actual survival. In fact, such a correlation has not been proven for most cancers. Often, when the doctor talks "response rate," the patients hear "cure." When these patients and their families learn that response rate does not often correlate with increased survival time or an improved quality of life, they begin to think the doctor has been lying to them. Although this chapter identifies the best combination of synergistic chemotherapeutic drugs are based on the response rate. It, by itself, is a poor parameter by which to determine its usually therapeutic benefits on advanced prostate cancer because it does not predict survival. Its effect on quality of life is usually determined by the nature of the treatment used.

Curative Chemotherapy

The intent of *curative chemotherapy* is to kill or destroy every last cancer cell lurking in your body. It involves shrinking and destroying the primary cancer and all measurable metastases, to produce a disease-free period of remission that is long enough that the patient will live out his normal life span. Unfortunately, while this goal might be true for some cancers, oncologists have not been able to achieve this goal in prostate cancer.

Complete Response

Complete response is the disappearance of all evidence of prostate cancer lasting for more than 28 days and a normalization of PSA level.

Partial Response

A partial response is a 50 percent or qreater reduction in measurably bidimensional disease lasting for 28 days or more.

Stabilized Disease

The disease results in less than a 50 percent regression in measurable tumor masses but not more than a 25 percent increase in all tumor masses.

Disease Progression

The disease results in a greater than 25 percent increase on the sum of the perpendicular diameters of all measurable masses or the appearance of new lesions.

Cytotoxic Chemotherapy

Drugs that are designed to kill cancer cells (but which can also kill healthy cells).

Increased Survival Time

A period of time added to the life of the patient due to treatment.

Understanding the Importance of a Randomized Clinical Trial (RCT)

To understand the claims made for chemotherapy, one must understand the reasons for a randomized clinical trials (RCT), or controlled trials. The chief reason for an RCT is to establish an objective basis to find out whether or not a drug works. If done properly, it offers a true measure of efficacy, time to progression, or survival. It is a human experiment in which the effect of one or more drugs is directly compared to that of another region given to patients with the same diagnoses. We would add that a secondary reason for RCT is to determine the synergistic relationship of two or more drugs in order to perfect a response rate that is able to benefit the highest number of patients for a given condition.

In the past, many patients made claims for treatments that were subject to misinterpretation, mistakes, or even fraud. Proof of the safety and effectiveness of a new drug was provided by testimonies from satisfied patients or their doctors, which were then published by drug manufacturers. Thus, the RCT is intended to eliminate the possibility of serous bias in studies of drugs.*

Hard Evidence

There are three kinds of studies that can provide hard evidence of a new drug's effectiveness.

1. *Randomized Comparisons of Patients Treated With a Drug versus Patients Not Treated with the Drug*

In such a study, the patient is assigned in advance to what is referred to as the study in a nondeliberate manner using a truly random mechanism. The "control" in such a study on patients with prostate cancer who receive either treatment or no treatment or receive a placebo, as a treatment with no substance.

2. *Randomized Comparison versus Immediate versus Different Chemotherapy*

Such a study attempts to determine whether chemotherapy should be given immediately or whether doctors should adopt a wait-and-see attitude, administering the drug only if the patient's symptoms worsen.

3. *Dose-Effect Studies*

In such a study, doctors attempt to find out whether higher doses of a drug cause an increase in survival time. Such studies must be carefully analyzed in order to prevent misinterpretation. Patients of different comparison should be avoided.

Soft Evidence

There are three kinds of studies that, while offering indirect proof, can provide useful information as to whether a drug is effective.

1. Randomized Comparisons of Two Chemotherapy Regimens

Patients are put into two groups, each one receiving a different combination of drugs. If one group of drugs proves much better than another, it can easily be construed that it will also be beneficial for patients. However, this might not be true. The difference between the two treatments may be due to more toxic treatment.

2. Nonrandomized Comparisons of Patient Groups

Nonrandomized means in essence that precautions have not been taken in assigning patients to the various groups of the study. As a result, all sorts of bias and subjective criteria can creep into the study.

3. Historical Trends

Data derived from historical trends are sometimes used as evidence of drug effectiveness. The effects of better treatments are sometimes reflected in national statistics on cancer mortality.

Determine The Effectiveness
of Chemotherapeutic Drugs

The PSA level, either used singly or in combination with other parameters, has come to be a significant factor in evaluating patient response to treatment. A significant decrease in the PSA level seems to be associated with improved survival when considering other factors. Dr. W. K. Kelly et al. investigated PSA as a measure of disease outcome in 110 hormone-refractory patients who had metastatic disease. Patients who had a decline in their PSA level equal to or greater than 50 percent had significantly longer median survival rate than did patients who had a less than 50 percent decline in PSA. As a result, the researchers concluded that a posttreatment PSA decline can be used as a surrogate endpoint to evaluate the effectiveness of new drugs.

By using the PSA level as an effectiveness indicator, it should allow a greater number of patients to be treated in clinical trials. A decline in PSA level is currently included as one criterion for disease response. However, the PSA is not yet established as an indicator of response or a measurement of disease outcome in metastatic prostate cancer patients. The response-rate criteria needs to be validated in phase III trials. Therefore, all prospective trials should compare a degree of PSA decline with response rate and survival in patients with metastatic disease should be ongoing. H. I. Scher, M.D. et al. indicated that a greater than 50 percent decline in PSA levels correlated with regression of measurable disease in only 67 percent of patients treated on a phase II clinical trial of trimetrexate. As a result, some investigators believe that a decline in PSA level of 80 percent should be the better criteria for judging chemotherapeutic drug effectiveness. Although it has been suggested that the PSA be used as a good marker for denoting response to treatment, it is not perfect; other parameters, such as the extent of the decline, the duration of decrease, and the time to reach nadir level, should also be considered.

Until recently, the results of most clinical trials involving cytotoxic chemotherapy treatments of metastatic prostate cancer patients have been disappointing to say the least. In 1988, M. A. Eisenberger, M.D., et al. reported that of 3,184 patients with metastatic prostate cancer who were treated with chemotherapy and reported in the literature, only 202 (6%) had complete and partial responses, while 485 (15%) had stabilized disease. In 1992, A. Yagodo, M.D., and and D. Petrylak, M.D., reviewed results of 26 drug trials evaluating single agents from 1987 to 1991 and found a similar trend. These trials had a response rate of 8.7 percent, indicating that chemotherapy fails to respond favorably to most cytotoxic agents. However, subsequent trials did show that by combining two or more drugs and changing the sequence of delivery, the doses did provide some patients with a higher response rate.

Different Approach to Improve the Response Rate

Although combinations of drugs have improved the response rate in several cases, combining two or more drugs is not the only way to achieve greater effectiveness. The following are three more approaches:

- Frequent dose intervals

  Some patients on chemotherapy have been known to improve the response rate by administering the drug over several intervals rather than in one interval.

- Dose intensification

  Sometimes, by increasing the dosage given to patients, the response rate may be increased. However, the "more is better" approach has not been shown to hold true for too many malignancies. There have been numerous studies in which the same combination of drugs was administered, but in different intensities, rates of administration, or time of administration. In some cases, the survival data was not indicated.

- Primary treatment followed by consideration in regimen

  In some instances, a patient receives a primary treatment followed by one or more drugs.

Treating Hormone-Refractory Prostate Cancer Patients With Chemotherapeutic Drugs

Although we have clinical evidence that PC SPES decreases the PSA level, we don't yet know the duration. Until we do, we must focus on chemotherapeutic drugs that provide the highest response rate to keep hormone-refractory patients alive as long as possible with a good quality of life. Initially, medical oncologists investigated several single drugs for metastatic prostate cancer patients. Unfortunately, toxicity has far outweighed any marginal benefit derived from single cytotoxic chemotherapy. In addition, almost all combination chemotherapeutics resulted in more frequent and more extreme toxicities than did a single agent for hormone-refractory prostate cancer, and benefits were marginal. Recently, physicians have had some promising results by combining certain single agents. For example, estramustine as a single agent has little activity in prostate cancer cell lines, but preclinical studies documented compelling evidence for synergy between estramustine and etoposide or vinblastine sulfate. The results led K. J. Pientz, M.D., et al. to conduct a phase II evaluation. The investigators treated 36 patients with oral estramustine 600 mg/day in daily divided doses. Overall, 52 percent of the patients experienced a 50 percent or greater reduction in PSA. Eighteen percent of patients with measurable soft tissue disease, 3 patients had a complete response and 6 patients had a partial response for a 50 percent response rate.

The following is a list of combination chemotherapeutic drugs that have resulted in one or more medical centers creating a combination of drugs that have rendered a 50 percent or better response rate.

Results with these drugs have indicated that some medical oncologists have not been able to duplicate a high response rate with the same combination of drugs as others. Consequently, it may be necessary for you as the patient to ask the medical oncologist to recommend the medical center where the high response rate is achieved.

The Best Combinations of Chemotherapy Drugs
With a Response Rate of 50 Percent or More

Drugs	Dose	Response Rate	PSA	Patients
• Estramustine day 1-42	600 mg/M IV	61%	decrease of greater than 50%	36
+ Vinblastine sulfate	4 mg/M IV weekly for 6 weeks			
• Estramustine	15 mg/M/day for 21 days	52%	decrease of greater than 50%	42
+ Ormetoposite	50 mg/m/day daily divided dose			
•				
• 5-FU	continuous infusion 250 mg/m^2	61%	decrease of greater than 50%	18
+ Doxorubicin	15 mg/m^2 weekly			
• Flosuridine (an analog of FU)	circadian infusion for 2 weeks and rest for 2 weeks	66%	decrease of greater than 60%	9
• Suramin	continuous infusion 350 mg/m^2/day	77%	50+	24

Drugs	Dose	Response Rate	PSA	Patients
• Stilphostrolut doxorubicin		63%	50	16
• Enzytaviablatine		63%	50	16
• Doxorubicin		57%	50	23
• Fam 5-Fluorooracilin Epirubicin + Mitomycin		50%	50	18
• Estramustine + Etoposide	15 mg/kg/ day for 21 days 50 mg/M^{2}d	50%	50	9
•				
• Faxol + Estramustine		50%	50	6
Estramustine + Taxol + Etoposite		52%		
• *Estramustine/Vinblastine* Ketoconazole		70%		
• Ketoconazole + Doxorubicin		63%		
• Estramustine + Docetaxel	280 mg administered one hour before and two hours after meals on day 1-5 plus 40-80 mg/m^2 on day Treatment repeated every 21 days.	63%		

Three Prominent Medical Oncologists Administering Combination Chemotherapy Drugs with High Response Rate

1. Dr. Daniel Petrylak
   Columbia Presbyterian Medical Center
   161 Fort Washington Ave.
   New York, NY 10032
   Phone: (212) 305-1731
   Fax: (212) 305-6762
   E-mail: dpp5@columbia.edu

2. Dr. Christopher Logothetis
   M.D. Anderson Cancer Treatment Center
   1515 Holcombe
   Houston, TX 77030
   Phone: (713) 792-2121; (713) 792-2830
   Fax: (713) 745-0827

3. Dr. Philip W. Kantoff
   44 Binney St.
   Dana Farber Cancer Institute
   Boston, MA 0211
   (617) 632-3466

Chapter 10

DEVELOPING A DIAGNOSTIC AND TREATMENT PLAN BY CONSIDERING THE "BESTS"

The intent of this chapter is to help you to devise a treatment plan base partially on what I have found through investigating scientific studies, clinical trials and investigational studies. Please be mindful that I am not a medical doctor. Therefore, consult your medical doctor prior to or during a conversation with your physician. If you have need of a study to share with your doctor, call the author at (516) 942-5000. A rationale for this book is to provide you with a source under one cover to enable you to do further research for agreeing or disagreeing what I have exposed under the cover of this book. I hope you will challenge me as well as your physician. Don't let your physicians discount what I have written about a particular test or treatment option. I am aware of too many physicians dispensing wrong information to patients.

Detecting Prostate Cancer

If it is suspected that you have prostate cancer and the sextant biopsy failed to detect it, ask your doctor to perform a 5-region biopsy.

Watchful Waiting

A key point to be realized is that an attempt should be made to kill the cancer tumor when it is small and at an early stage. If you are waiting to do more research before making a treatment decision, you should consider following options:

First: Do nothing.

Second: Undergo CHT for six months to get your PSA below 4.0 ng/ml.

Third: Take two to three capsules of PC SPES daily, take 400 mg. three times a day plus 400 mg of garlic five times a day to prevent a possible blood clot.

Fourth: Undergo an antiandrogen and Proscar. Monitor your PSA with the ultrasensitive PSA.

Fifth: Take chemoprevention vitamins, minerals, and supplements, go on an exercise program, make life style changes and take two capsules of PC SPES and vitamin E and garlic.

Sixth: Monitor your PSA with the ultrasensitive PSA.

Radical Prostatectomy

The single most point you should realize is that if your are opting for surgery the cancer should be confined to the capsule. Consider a treatment plan consisting of the following:

First: Undergo a spectroscopic MRI (MRSI).

Second: Use one of the top three surgeons in the country to perform the operation.

Third: Use the ultrasensitive PSA to monitor your disease post treatment.

Fourth: Make a list of the possible chemoprevention vitamins, minerals and other agents, go on an exercise program, make appropriate lifestyle changes. Add two capsules of PC SPES, 400 mg vitamin E three times a day and two capsules of PC SPES to prevent a recurrence.

Fifth: Continue to monitor your PSA with the ultrasensitive PSA.

If you should have a recurrence of prostate cancer (PSA above .02ng/ml), initiate the following steps:

First: Get another MRSI to decide if your prostate cancer is still organ confined.

Second: If your disease is still organ confined, consider the following treatment options:

      • Contact the clinics in Georgia to determine if you are eligible to receive the prostRcision. Dr. Critz has performed seed implantations and external beam radiation on nearly a hundred failed radical prostatectomy patients.

or

- Contact a physician who will perform a combination of hormonal therapy and external beam radiation.

or

- Undergo an antiandrogen and Proscar.

Third: Monitor your retreatment with an ultrasensitive PSA.

Fourth: Undergo some of the best combination/intermittent hormonal therapy.

External Beam Radiation

If you opted for external beam radiation, you should consider the following:

First: Simultaneously undergo external beam radiation and three years of combination hormonal therapy (CHT).

Second: Monitor your PSA with the ultrasensitive PSA test. You and your physician will need to decide jointly on an ultrasensitive PSA level to determine a recurrence of prostate cancer.

Third: Undergo two capsules of PC SPES three times a day, 400 mg of vitamin E three times a day and 400 mg of garlic three times a day.

- Undergo CHT for six months, then discontinue the CHT and go on three capsules of PC SPES at bed time.

Fourth: If you should get a recurrence take CHT for several months to reduce your PSA level below 4.0 ng/ml, then discontinue the CHT and undergo three capsules of PC SPES at night with the blood thinning supplements.

Fifth: Monitor your PSA with an ultrasensitive PSA on a monthly basis.

Sixth: If the PC SPES fails, undergo CHT as long as possible or another viable complementary treatment.

Seventh: Undergo certain synergetic chemotherapeutic drugs.

Seed Implantation

If you opted for seed implantation, consider the following:

First: Check to see if your disease has invaded the lymph nodes by getting a laparoscopic lymph node dissection.

Second: If the disease has not, undergo a prostRcision.

Third: Monitor your PSA with an ultrasensitive PSA six months after treatment and monthly thereafter.

Fourth: Establish a list of possible chemoprevention supplements, a list of vitamins, minerals, go on an exercise program, make some life style changes, undergo two capsules of PC SPES, 400 mg of vitamin E three times a day and 400 mg of garlic five times a day.

Fifth: If you should have a recurrence and the disease is localized, undergo a retreatment of seeds.

Sixth: Continue to monitor your PSA with an ultrasensitive PSA.

Combination Hormonal Therapy (CHT)

If you opted or are currently undergoing CHT, consider the following:

First: Take CHT for six months, discontinue the CHT and commence to take three capsules of PC SPES at night and 400 mg of vitamin E three times a day and 400 mg of garlic five times a day.

Second: Monitor your PSA monthly.

Third: If you get a recurrence of prostate cancer, go back on either CHT or intermittent CHT.

Fourth: If and when CHT is not working, undergo the best synergetic drugs.

PC SPES Caps

If you opted for PC SPES, consider the following options:

First: Undergo two capsules of PC SPES three times a day until a "threshold level" is determined. Also, take 400 mg of vitamin E three times a day plus 400 mg of garlic five times a day.

Second: Take combination hormone therapy (CHT) or Honovan until your PSA declines below three. Discontinue the CHT and begin the PC SPES with the blood thinning supplements.

Third: If the PC SPES should fail, consider the following:

> 1. Go back on CHT.
>
> or
>
> 2. Go on Vitae Elixxir.
>
> or
>
> 3. Go on a combination of drugs cited in this book.

How You May Use This Information

To become more familiar with prostRcision, do the following:

1. Request the clinic to send you information on Dr. Frank A. Critz's satisfied study.

2. Visit the clinic's website at http:\\www.prostrcision.com/pages/faq.html.

3. Request the clinic to forward to you its brochure on prostRcision.

4. If possible, visit the clinic to observe the treatment and the humanistic manner in which the administrative staff treats patients and the professionalism of the medical center.

5. Engage in a conversation with patients who have undergone the treatment.

Appendix

PSA Nadir Level: The Test Result That Determines Cure

The PSA nadir test is the single most important test made after any treatment for prostate cancer. It is far more important than pretreatment PSA, Gleason score, or stage. The PSA nadir test determines whether or not a man will be cured of prostate cancer.

The PSA nadir is the lowest PSA reading achieved after any treatment for prostate cancer. This includes any radiation technique (e.g., seed implantation, conformal beam radiation, proton beam radiation, prostRcision), radical prostatectomy and cryosurgery. Every man treated for prostate cancer should know his PSA nadir.

Only men have a prostate gland, and PSA is produced only by prostate cells, both normal and cancerous, but not by any other cell. In contrast, women do not have a prostate gland. If you performed a PSA test on a woman, you would not find any.

Also, prostate cancer cells produce PSA no matter where they are located. Prostate cancer cells inside the prostate, those that have penetrated the capsule, and those that have metastasized to bone all manufacture PSA equally well.

To illustrate how the PSA nadir works, let's imagine that a man has been diagnosed with stage T1C prostate cancer, has undergone a radical prostatectomy, and has been cured. When the surgery was performed, the prostate gland (all normal prostate cells) was removed, and since the man was cured, all prostate cancer cells would have been removed also. Thus, there would be no prostate cells left in this man. Therefore there would be no prostate cells to make PSA. His PSA would have quickly fallen to an undetectable level after surgery. Since the PSA nadir is the lowest PSA reached, we would say this man has achieved an *undetectable PSA nadir* and that he has been potentially cured of prostate cancer by radical prostatectomy. Note the word *potentially*.

The actual PSA number that means an undetectable PSA is found in cure-rate calculations after radical prostatectomy in research papers published in medical journals. Dr. Patrick Walsh uses a PSA nadir 0.2 ng/ml or lower to indicate an undetectable PSA when he reports cure rates.

But what happens when a PSA nadir of 0.2 ng/ml or lower is not achieved after radical prostatectomy? If the PSA is still detectable, then prostate cancer cells were left behind. *Detectable PSA* (above 0.2 ng/ml) after surgery guarantees that a patient is not cured.

As you can see, if a PSA of 0.2 ng/ml or lower is achieved after surgery, the patient has been potentially cured. But if the PSA is more than 0.2, the man still has prostate cancer.

Achieving 0.2 ng/ml or lower after surgery, however does not guarantee a cure. It is only the first step toward cure. There is a second step: the PSA nadir of 0.2 ng/ml must be achieved and must stay at 0.2—or lower—forever. From a practical standpoint, it should stay at that level for at least 10 years after surgery.

Suppose a man has achieved a PSA level of 0.2 ng/ml (or lower) after a radical prostatectomy. Now, let's assume that a tiny amount of microscopic cancer cells were left behind. Although these cells produce PSA, there are not enough of them to manufacture a detectable amount immediately after surgery. However, as time passes, these cells will multiply, and eventually there will be enough of them to produce enough PSA to cause the PSA level to rise above 0.2 ng/ml.

The rate at which prostate cancer grows varies considerably. Some cancer cells multiply rapidly, and more than 0.2 ng/ml of PSA can be found only a few months after surgery. Other cancer cells multiply slowly and require several years to produce a detectable PSA. Almost all cancer cells left behind after surgery will produce a detectable amount of PSA within 10 years of treatment, although a few of Dr. Walsh's patients have had a recurrence after more than 10 years.

Using the PSA nadir test, the cure rates for radical prostatectomy can be calculated. Cure of prostate cancer is defined as the percent of treated men who achieved and maintained a PSA nadir of 0.2 ng/ml or lower 10 years after surgery. The radical-prostatectomy medical study most commonly quoted is from Johns Hopkins University, with surgery performed by Dr. Patrick Walsh. Dr. Walsh's 10-year cure rate is 68 percent. This means that of every 100 men who had a radical prostatectomy, 68 achieved and maintained an undetectable PSA nadir of 0.2 ng/ml or less for 10 years after surgery. This also means that 32 out of 100 either never achieved PSA nadir 0.2 ng/ml or achieved this level for less than 10 years.

PSA Nadir After Radiotherapy of Prostate Cancer

In contrast to surgery, the prostate gland is still present after radiotherapy of prostate cancer. Therefore, you might think that use of the PSA nadir test would be different after radiation. That is not true.

For men to be cured with radiotherapy, an undetectable PSA nadir (0.2 ng/ml or lower) must be achieved and maintained after treatment. If a PSA nadir of 0.2 ng/ml is not achieved, or if it is not maintained, men will not be cured of prostate cancer by radiotherapy except under rare circumstances. This principle applies to any form of radiation—prostRcision, seed implant alone, conformal beam radiation, proton beam radiation, and so on.

The only difference between radiotherapy and radical prostatectomy is the time it takes after treatment to achieve a PSA level of 0.2 ng/ml. When a radical prostatectomy is performed, both normal prostate cells and hopefully all cancer cells are removed immediately. The PSA should reach an undetectable nadir within 6 weeks of surgery.

However, after radiotherapy, it takes time for normal prostate cells and cancer cells to die and disintegrate. Death of these cells is indicated by a falling PSA level after treatment. The median time to achieve 0.2 ng/ml after radiotherapy is 27 months. The death rate of normal prostate cells and cancerous prostate cells varies considerably, but the cure rate is unrelated to how fast these cells die.

The finding that a PSA nadir of 0.2 ng/ml or lower is required after radiotherapy of prostate cancer is based on measuring the PSA nadir that was achieved and maintained by men cured of prostate cancer by radiation. Dr. Critz's group was the first group to find the relationship between PSA nadir and cure with radiation. Almost all research on PSA nadir after radiotherapy for prostate cancer has been performed by doctors at Radiotherapy Clinics of Georgia in men treated with prostRcision. They have had four peer-reviewed research papers published on this subject, the first in 1995. Additionally, they have presented their findings at all major peer-reviewed medical meetings: the American Urological Association (AUA), American Society of Clinical Oncology (ASCO), American Radium Society (ARS), and American Brachytherapy Society (ABS). Their last peer-reviewed research paper was published in the *Journal of Urology* in April 1999.

In their initial research in 1995, Dr. Critz's group showed that the PSA nadir goal for cure of prostate cancer by radiotherapy was 0.5 ng/ml. However, they noted that most men's PSA fell to much lower levels. Dr. Critz's group reanalyzed all their data in preparation for the May 1999 meeting of the American Urological Association (AUA) in Dallas, Texas, where their findings were presented. Dr. Critz conclusively showed that to be cured of prostate cancer by irradiation, with few exceptions, a man must achieve and maintain a PSA nadir of 0.2 ng/ml or lower. He showed that of all men cured with prostRcision using the new, high-dose ultrasound-guided implant method, 97 percent achieved and maintained a PSA nadir of 0.2 ng/ml or lower. Only 3 percent of cured men had a PSA nadir of 0.3 to 1.0 ng/ml. None with a PSA nadir above 1.0 ng/ml were cured. Dr. Critz concluded that cure-rate calculations for radiotherapy of prostate cancer should be done using a PSA nadir of 0.2 ng/ml. He also noted that most men who achieved 0.2 ng/ml or less actually achieved 0.1 ng/ml or less. However, measuring 0.1 ng/ml requires a special PSA test.

Urologists use a PSA nadir of 0.2 ng/ml to determine cure after radical prostatectomy. Therefore, the definition of cure for radiotherapy of prostate cancer is identical to that after surgery: men must achieve and maintain an undetectable PSA nadir, meaning 0.2 ng/ml or less, for 10 or more years after treatment. These findings should apply to any radiotherapy method.

The identical PSA nadir goal for both prostRcision and radical prostatectomy indicates that all prostate cells, both normal and cancerous, are destroyed by prostRcision just as effectively as having them surgically removed by a radical prostatectomy. In other words, if you give enough radiation to cure prostate cancer, all, or virtually all, normal prostate cells are also destroyed. The dose of radiation needed to cure prostate cancer is more than what normal prostate cells can tolerate. Remember with prostRcision, the dose of radiation inside the prostate is intensified by giving conformal beam radiation after the iodine seed implant since both normal and cancer cells are irradiated simultaneously.

If you think about it, a "prostatectomy" is performed by prostRcision, just as is done with surgery, except that the muscles that control urination and the sex nerves are not removed with prostRcision. The word *prostRcision* is derived from this concept, since prostRcision means "excision of the prostate with radiation."

These findings may also explain why the cure rate for prostRcision is so high. If you leave normal prostate cells behind after radiation, what is to prevent them from making more prostate cancer? However, if you destroy all normal and cancerous prostate cells, you will prevent a man from getting any new cancer.

These findings from the Radiotherapy Clinics of Georgia—that patients need to achieve and maintain a PSA nadir of 0.2 ng/ml after radiotherapy—have not been popular with doctors in the United States who treat prostate cancer by other radiotherapy methods. These doctors believe that an undetectable PSA nadir is too strict for radiotherapy. They are afraid that calculating cure rates with an undetectable PSA nadir will lower their cure-rate claims.

These other doctors believe that you can destroy 100 percent of all prostate cancer cells, but that normal prostate cells, which are located next to cancer cells inside the prostate, will not be bothered very much by radiation and will keep on making normal amounts of PSA. This is not logical. No research paper has ever been published to back up the belief that normal cells remain after destroying all cancer cells with radiation. It is much more reasonable to believe that if you give enough radiation to destroy prostate cancer cells, you also destroy all, or virtually all, normal cells. All peer-reviewed research papers show this.

Achieving PSA Nadir After prostRcision

After treatment with prostRcision, prostate cancer cells, as well as normal cells, begin to die and disintegrate. The death of normal and cancerous prostate cells can be measured by using the PSA test. The goal is to achieve a PSA nadir of 0.2 ng/ml, which represents an undetectable PSA, and for all men this is achieved at a median time of 27 months after the implant.

Table 7-1 shows how the PSA falls at each follow-up visit.

The PSA measurements in the table are median PSA levels. This means that half the men in each PSA group have a PSA lower than and half have a PSA higher than each PSA measurement. For example, the median PSA is 2.0 ng/ml at 6-month follow-up for men with a PSA of more than 20.0 ng/ml before treatment. Therefore, half of the men at 6-month follow-up had a PSA of less than 2.0, and half had a PSA more than 2.0. This means that some cancers die quickly and others slowly.

Although we may think that achieving a low PSA nadir rapidly is better, in fact that is not correct. Men treated with prostRcision were divided into "fast PSA fallers" and "slow PSA fallers." The cure rate for slow fallers and fast fallers is identical. The rate of fall of PSA does not make any

Table 7-1. PSA After prostRcision

Month after Implant	Pretreatment PSA Group			
	NG/ML			
	<4.0	4.1–10.0	10.1–20.0	>20.0
3 Mo.	1.2	1.8	2.6	3.7
6 Mo.	0.8	1.1	1.6	2.0
12 Mo.	0.5	0.6	0.8	0.9
18 Mo.	0.4	0.5	0.7	0.6
24 Mo.	0.4	0.3	0.5	0.5
30 Mo.	0.2	0.2	0.2	0.4
36 Mo.	0.2	0.2	0.2	0.2
42 Mo.	0.1	0.1	0.1	0.1

difference in terms of curing prostate cancer with prostRcision. It is not a race to see who crosses the finish line first. You are a winner no matter when you cross it. The finish line is achieving a PSA nadir of 0.2 ng/ml or less.

Cure Rate According To PSA Nadir Achieved

Regardless of whether man is treated with radiation or surgery, the PSA nadir achieved is the single most important factor that determines whether he will be cured of prostate cancer. The cure rates, according to PSA nadir achieved after prostRcision, are given in the table below. Cure is directly related to how low the PSA nadir goes. These cure rates were calculated for men treated with prostRcision using both the old, low-dose, open implant method and the new, high-dose transperineal method. None of the men in these calculations ever took hormones.

PSA Nadir Achieved	10-Year Cure Rate
(ng/ml)	
0.2 or less	92%
0.3 to 1.0	41%
more than 1.0	0%

However, for men treated by prostRcision using the new transperineal implant method, the 5-year cure rate is 98 percent for those men who achieve a PSA nadir of 0.2 ng/ml. Furthermore, if a PSA nadir of 0.2 ng/ml is achieved, it does not make any difference what the pretreatment PSA was or the Gleason score or the stage.

PSA Bounce

PSA bounce causes a great deal of anxiety in men. After prostRcision, 31 percent of men have a PSA bounce.

What is PSA bounce? Think of PSA after treatment as an airplane that is descending to land at an airport. The airport is the PSA nadir of 0.2 ng/ml or lower. On a windless day, the airplane will smoothly come in for a landing. Now think of an airplane landing on a windy day. While descending to land, a gust of wind comes underneath the plane causing it to bounce up temporarily and then fall back into its flight path to the airport.

This analogy describes what is meant by PSA bounce. Out of every three men treated, one will have a progressive fall in PSA but it will bounce upward on one or more occasions and then return to fall to 0.2 ng/ml. The most common time for a PSA bounce to occur is between the 12- and 24-month follow-up, but a PSA bounce can occur at any time. For example, 1 percent of men have a PSA bounce at the 3-month follow-up. PSA bounce is thought to be due to irritation inside the prostate gland, which causes an excessive leakage of PSA into the bloodstream where PSA is measured.

When a bounce occurs, the average rise in the PSA is 0.4 ng/ml. However, bounces as high as 16 ng/ml have been seen. PSA bounce is uncommonly seen when the PSA is above 4.0 ng/ml before bounce. It is very rarely seen when the PSA has fallen to 0.2 ng/ml or less. Since a PSA of 0.2 ng/ml indicates that all cells have been destroyed, there are no cells to cause a bounce.

PSA bounce frightens men when it occurs. It is the most common reason that men call the doctors at RCOG after they have been treated. But PSA bounce has no impact on being cured except in a very odd way: men who have a PSA bounce have a higher cure rate than do men who never had a PSA bounce.

References

Chapter 1 References:

Adlercreutz H., H. Honjo, A. Higashi, T. Fotsis, E. Hamalainen, T. Hasegawa, and H. Okada. "Urinary Excretion of Lignans and Isoflavonoid Phytoestrogens in Japanese Men and Women Consuming a Traditional Japanese Diet." *American Journal of Clinical Nutrition* 54(6) (1991): 1093–1100.

Agarwal, K.C. "Therapeutic Actions of Garlic Constituents." *Med Res Rev* 16 (1996): 111–24.

Ahmad, N. et al. "Green Tea Constituent, Epigallocatechin-3-gallate and Induction of Apoptosis and Cell Cycle Arrest in Human Carcinoma Cells." *Journal of the National Cancer Institute* 89 (1997): 1881–86.

Akiyama, T. et al. "Genistein, a Specific Inhibitor of Tyrosine-Specific Protein Kinases." *Journal of Biologic Chemistry* 262 (1987): 5592–95.

"The Alpha-Tocopherol, Beta Carotene Cancer Prevention Study Group. The effect of vitamin E and beta carotene on the incidence of lung cancer and other cancers in male smokers." *New England Journal of Medicine* 330 (1994): 1029–35.

Boone, C.W., G.J. Kelloff, and V.E. Steele. "Natural History of Intraepithelial Neoplasia in Humans with Implications for Cancer Chemoprevention Strategy." *Cancer Research* 52 (1992): 1651–59.

Bostwick, D. G. "Target Populations and Strategies for Chemoprevention Trials of Prostate Cancer," *Journal of Cellular Biochemistry* Suppl., 19 (1994): 191.

Carter, H.B. and D.S. Coffey. "The Prostate: An Increasing Medical Problem." *Prostate* 16 (1990): 39–48.

Carter, H.B., S. Piantadose, and J.T. Isaacs. "Clinical Evidence for and Implications of the Multistep Development of Prostate Cancer." *Journal of Urology* 143 (1990): 742–46.

Clark, L.C., G.F. Combs, Jr., B.W. Turnbull, E.H. Slate, D.K. Chalker, and J. Chow et al. "Effects of Selenium Supplementation for Cancer Prevention in Patients With Carcinoma of the Skin. A randomized controlled trial. Nutritional Prevention of Cancer Study Group." *JAMA* 276: 1957–63, 1996.

Colditz, G.A., L.G. Branch, and R.J. Lipnick et al. "Increased Green and Yellow Vegetable Intake and Lowered Cancer Deaths in an Elderly Population." *American Journal of Clinical Nutrition* 41 (1985): 32–6.

Dorant, E. et al. "Consumption of Onions and a Reduced Risk of Stomach Carcinoma." *Gastroenterology* 110 (1996): 12–20.

El-Bayoumy, K. "The Role of Selenium in Cancer Prevention." In: V.T. DeVita, S. Hellman, and S.S. Rosenberg eds. *Practice of Oncology.* 4th ed. Philadelphia: J. B. Lippincott, 1991: 1–15.

Feldman, D. et al. "Vitamin D: Metabolism and Action." In: R. Marcus, D. Feldman, J. Kelsey eds. *Osteoporosis.* San Diego: Academic Press, 1996: 205–35.

Folkman, J. "What is the Evidence That Tumors are Angiogenesis-Dependent?" *Journal National Cancer Institute* 82 (1990): 4–6.

Fotsis, T., M. Pepper, H. Aldercruetz, G. Fleischmann, T. Haases, R. Montesano, and L. Schweigerer. "Genistein, a Dietary-Derived Inhibitor of In Vitro Angiogenesis." Proceedings of the National Academy of Science, USA 90 (1993): 2690–94.

Fujiki, H., A. Komori, and M. Suganuma. "Chemoprevention of Cancer." In: G.T. Bowden and S.M Fischer eds. *Comprehensive Toxicology: Chemical Carcinogenesis & Anticarcinogens.* Oxford, England: Elsevier Science, Ltd. (in press).

Fujiki H., S. Yoshizawa, and T. Horiuchi et al. "Anticarcinogenic Effects of (-)-Epigallocatechin Gallate." *Prev Medicine* 21 (1992): 503–9.

Giovannucci, E., A. Ascherio, E. B. Rimm, M. J. Stampfer, G. A. Colditz, and W. C. Willett. "Intake of Carotenoids and Retinol in Relation to Risk of Prostate Cancer." *Journal of the National Cancer Institute*, Vol. 87, No. 23 (December 6, 1995): 1767–76.

Harras, A., ed. *Cancer Rates and Risks*, 4th ed. 1996.

Heinonen, O.P. et al. "Prostate Cancer and Supplementation With Alpha-Tocopherol and Beta Carotene; Incidence and Mortality in a Controlled Trial." *Journal of the National Cancer Institute* 90 (1998): 440–46.

Helzlsouer, K.J., G.W. Comstock, and J.S. Morris. "*Selenium, Lycopene, a*-Tocopherol, *b*-Carotene and Subsequent Bladder Cancer." *Cancer Research* 49 (1989): 895–900.

Herman, C. et al. "Soybean Phytoestrogen Intake and Cancer Risk." *Journal of Nutrition* 125 (1995): 757S–770S. Efficacious use of food resources in the United States. USDA. Technical Bulletin number 963, from the US Government Printing Office, Washington, DC.

Heshmat, M.Y., L. Kaul, J. Lovi, M.A. Jackson, A.G. Jackson, and G.W. Jones et al. "Nutrition and Prostate Cancer: A Case-Control Study." *Prostate* 6 (1985): 7–17.

Hirayama, T. "A Large Scale Cohort Study on Cancer Risks with Special Reference to the Risk Reducing Effects of Green-Yellow Vegetable Consumption." *Ins Symp Princess Takamatsu Cancer Res Fund* 16 (1985): 41–53.

Holick, M. F. "Vitamin D Biosynthesis, Metabolism, and Mode of Action." In: L. J. DeGroot ed. *Endocrinology*. New York: Grune and Stratton, 1989. 902–26.

Horoszewicz, J.S., S.S. Leong, and E. Kawinski et al. "LNCaP Model of Human Prostatic Carcinoma." *Cancer Research* 43 (1983): 1809–18.

Howie, B.J. and T.D. Shultz. "Dietary and Hormonal Interrelationships Among Vegetarian Seventh-Day Adventists and Non-Vegetarian Men." *American Journal Clinical Nutrition* 42 (1985): 127–34.

Imoto M., T. Yamashit, H. Swaw, S. Kusaswa, H. Naganawa, T. Takeuch, Z. Boa-quan and K. Umezawa. "Inhibition of Cellular Phosphatidylinositol Turnover by Psi-Tectorigenin." *FEBS Lett* 230 (1988): 43–46.

Ip, C. "The Chemopreventive Role of Selenium in Carcinogenesis." *Journal of American coll Toxicol.* 5 (1986): 7–20.

Isaacs, J.T., W.B. Isaacs, and W.F. Feitz, et al. "Establishment and Characterization of Seven Dunning Rat Prostatic Cancer Cell Lines and Their Use in Developing Methods for Predicting Metastatic Abilities of Prostatic Cancers." *Prostate* 9 (1986): 261–281.

Knekt, P., A. Aromaa, J. Maatela, G. Alfthan, R.K. Aaran, and M. Hakama, et al. "Serum Selenium and Subsequent Risk of Cancer Among Finnish Men and Women." *Journal National Cancer Institute* 82 (1990): 864–8.

Kohn, E.C.: "Development and prevention of metastasis." *Anticancer Research* 13 (1993): 2552–2559.

Kolonel, L. N. et al. "Relationship of Dietary Vitamin A and Ascorbic Acid Intake to the Risk of Cancers of the Lung, Bladder and Prostate In Hawaii." *National Cancer Institute Monograph* 68 (1985): 137–142.

Kroes, R., R.B. Beems, M.C. Bosland, G.S.J. Brennik, and E.J. Sinkeldam. "Nutritional Factors in Lung, Colon and Prostate Carcinogenesis in Animal Models." *Federal Proceedings* 45 (1986): 136–41.

Kyle, E. et al. "Genistein-Induced Apoptosis of Prostate Cancer Cells is Preceded by a Specific Decrease in Focal Adhesion Kinase Activity." *Molecular Pharmacology* 51 (1997): 193–200.

Lau, B.H.S., P.P. Tadi, J.M. and Tosk. "Allium Sativum (Garlic) and Cancer Prevention." *Nutrition Research* 10 (1990): 937–48.

Levy, J., E. Bosin, and B. Feldman, et al. *Nutrition and Cancer* 24 (1995): 257–66.

Lippman, S. M., S. E. Benner, and W. Ki Hong. "Cancer Chemoprevention." *Journal Clinical Oncology* 12 (1994): 851–73.

Maik, H., and M. Pilat et al. "Inhibition of In Vitro Tumor Cell-Endothelial Adhesion by Modified Citrus Pectin: A Ph Modified Natural Complex Carbohydrate." Proceedings Annual Meeting American Association Cancer Research, 36 (1995): A377.

Maramag, C. et al. "Effect of Vitamin C on Prostate Cancer Cells In Vitro: Effect on Cell Number, Viability and DNA Synthesis." Prostate 32 (1997): 188, 195.

Mills, P. K. et al. "Cohort Study of Diet, Lifestyle and Prostate Cancer in Adventist Men." Cancer 64 (1989): 598–604.

Milner, J. A. "Garlic: Its Anticarcinogenic and Antitumorigenic Properties." Nutritional Review 54 (1996): S82–86.

Mitscher L.A., S.P. Pillai, and D.M. Shankel. "Naturally Occurring Antimutagenic and Cytoprotective Agents." Presented at the American Chemical Society. June 1997.

Nomura, A.M., and L.N. Kolonel. "Prostate Cancer: A Current Perspective." Epidemiological Review 13 (1991): 200–27.

Okura, A., H. Arakawa, H. Oka, T. Yoshinara, and Y. Monden. "Effect of Genistein on Topoisomerase Activity and Growth of (Val 12) Ha-Ras-Transformed NIH 3T3 Cells." Biochem Biophys Res Commun. 157 (1988): 183–89.

Pienta, K.J. and P.S. Esper. "Risk Factors for Prostate Cancer." Ann Intern Med 118 (1993): 793–803.

Pinto, J. and R. S. Rivlin. "Garlic Constituents Modify Expression of Biomarkers for Human Prostatic Carcinoma Cells." FASEB Journal 11 (Feb. 28 1997): A439.

Pinto, J. T. and R. S. Rivlin. "Garlic and Prevention of Prostate Cancer." In P. Lachance and H. Pierson, eds. Designer Foods III. Westport, Conn.: Food and Nutrition Press. In press.

Platt, D. and A. Raz. "Modulation of the Lung Colonization of B16-F1 Melanoma Cells by Citrus Pectin," Journal of National Cancer Institute, 84 (1992): 438–42.

Potter, J. D. and K. Steinmetz. "Vegetables, Fruit, and Phytoestrogens as Preventative Agents." IARC Science Publications 139 (1996): 61–90.

Raz, A. and R. Lotan. "Endogenous Galactoside-Binding Lectins: A New Class of Functional Tumor Cell Surface Molecules Related to Metastasis." *Cancer Metastasis Review,* 6 (1987): 433–52.

Ripple, M.O., W.F. Henry, R.P. Rag, and G. Wilding. "Pro-oxidant-Antioxidant Shift Induced by Androgen Treatment of Human Prostate Carcinoma Cells." *Journal of National Cancer Institute* 89 (1997): 40–48.

Schwartz, G. G. et al. "Is Vitamin D Deficiency a Risk Factor for Prostate Cancer?" (Hypothesis) *Anticancer Research* 10 (1990): 1307–12.

Spallholz, J. "On the Nature of Selenium Toxicity and Carcinostatic Activity." *Free Radical Biology and Medicine* 17 (1994): 45–64.

Sporn, M. B. "Approaches to Prevention of Epithelial Cancer During The Preneoplastic Period." *Cancer Research* 36 (1976): 2699.

Sporn, M. B., N. M. Dunlop, and D. L. Newton. "Prevention of Chemical Carcinogenesis by Vitamin A and its Synthetic Analogs (Retinoids)." *Federal Proceedings* 35, (1976): 1332–38.

Takai, K. "Promotional Effects of High-Fat Diet on Chemical Carcinogenesis of the Prostate." *Japanese Journal of Urology* 82 (1991): 871–80.

Talamini, R., S. Franceschi, C. La Vecchia, D. Serraino, S. Barra, and E. Negri. "Diet and Prostatic Cancer: A Case-Control Study in Northern Italy." *Nutrition and Cancer* 18 (1992): 277–86.

Taylor, P.R. and D. Albanes. "Selenium, Vitamin E, and Prostate Cancer—Ready for Prime Time?" *Journal of the National Cancer Institute,* Vol. 90, No. 16, (August 19, 1998).

Wang, L. and E.C. Hammond. "Lung Cancer, Fruit, Green Salad, and Vitamin Pills." *Chinas Medical Journal* 98 (1985): 206–10.

Wei, H., L. Wei, R. Bowen, K. Frenkel, and S. Barnes. "Inhibition of Tumor Promoter-Induced Hydrogen Perioxide Production In Vitro and In Vivo by Genistein." *Nutrition and Cancer* 20 (1) (1993): 1–12.

Whanger, P. et al. "Metabolism of Subtoxic Levels of Selenium in Animals and Humans." *Annals of Clinical and Laboratory Science* 26 (1996): 99–113.

Yoshizawa, S., T. Horiuchi, H. Fujiki, T. Yoshida, T. Okuda, and T. Sugimura. "Antitumor Promoting Activity of (-_- Epigallocatechin Gallate, the Main Constituent Of 'Tanin' in Green Tea." *Phytother Research* 1 (1987): 44–7.

Yu, W., D.W. Warren, X. Heston, and W.D. Fair. "Soy Isoflavones Decrease the High-Fat Promoted Growth of Human Prostate Cancer: Results of In Vitro and Animal Studies." *Proceedings of American Urology Association* 153 (1995): 269A (Abstract No. 161).

Zhang, G. and E.E. Fraley. "Continuous Sinusoidal Infusion of Floxuridine (FUDR) for Treatment of Hormonal Refractory Metastatic Prostate Cancer." *Proceedings American Soc Clinical Oncology* 9 (1990): 419.

Zigler, R.G. "Vegetables, Fruit and Carotenoids and the Risk of Cancer." *American Journal of Clinical Nutrition* 53 (1991): 2515–95.

Chapter 2 References:

Carter, H.G.B., J.D. Pearson, and J. Metter et al. "Longitudinal Evaluation Of Prostate Specific Antigen Levels in Men with and Without Prostate Disease." *JAMA* 167 (1992): 2215.

Catalona, W.J., D.S. Smith, and T.L. Ratcliff et al. "Measurement of Prostate Specific Antigen in Serum as a Screening Test for Prostate Cancer." *New England Journal of Medicine* 324 (1991): 1156.

Cooner, W.H., B.R. Mosley, and C.L. Rutherford Jr. et al. "Prostate Cancer Detection in a Clinical Urological Practice by Ultrasonograph, Digital Rectal Examination and Prostate Specific Antigen." *Journal of Urology* 143 (1990): 1146.

Graves, H.C.B., N. Wehner, and T.A. Stamey. "Ultra-Sensitive Radioimmunoassay for Prostate Specific Antigen." *Clinical Chem* 38 (1992): 735.

Osterling, J.E., and P.C. Walsh et al. "Prostate Specific Antigen in the Preoperative and Postoperative Evaluation of Localized Prostatic Cancer Treated with Radical Prostatectomy." *Journal of Urology* 139 (1988): 766.

Schmid, P.P., J.E. McNeal, and T.A. Stamey. "Observations on the Doubling Time of Prostate Cancer. The Use of Serial PSA in Patients with Untreated Disease as a Measure of Increasing Cancer Volume." *Cancer* 71 (1993): 2031.

Sensabaugh, G.F. "Isolation and Characterization of a Semen-Specific Protein from Human Semial Plasma. A Potential, New Marker for Semen Identification." *Journal of Forensic Science* 23 (1978): 106.

Stamey, T.A., H.C.B. Graves, and N. Hefner et al. "Early Detection of Residual Prostate Cancer After Radical Prostatectomy by an Ultrasensitive Assay for Prostate Specific Antigen." *Journal of Urology* 149 (1993): 787.

Stamey, T.A., J.N. Kabalin, M. Ferrari, and N. Yang. "Prostate Specific Antigen in the Diagnosis and Treatment of Adenocarcinoma of the Prostate IV. Anti-Androgen Treated Patients." *Journal of Urology* 141 (1989): 1088.

Stamey, T.A., J.N. Kabalin, and J.E. McNeal et al. "Prostate specific Antigen in the Diagnosis and Treatment of Adenocarcinoma of the Prostate II. Radical Prostatectomy Treated Patients." *Journal of Urology* 141 (1989): 1076.

Stamey, T.A., N. Yang, and A.R. Hay et al. "Prostate Specific Antigen as a Serum Marker for Adenocarcinoma of the Prostate." *New England Journal of Medicine* 317 (1987): 909.

Vessela, R.L., J. Noteboom, and P.H. Kange. "Evaluation of Automated Abbott IMX Prostate Specific Antigen (PSA) Immunoassay." *Clin Chem* 38 (1992): 2044.

Chapter 3 References:

Bartolozzi, C., I. Menchi, R. Lencioni, S. Semi, A. Lapini, G. Barbanti, A. Bozza, A. Amorosi, A. Manganelli, and M. Carim. "Local Staging of Prostate Carcinoma with Endorectal Coil MRI: Correlation with Whole-Mount Radical Prostatectomy Specimens." *European Radiology* 6 (1996): 339–45.

Bessette, A., U.G. Mueller-Lisse, M. Swanson, D.V. Vigneron, J. Scheidler, A. Srivastava, P. Wood, H. Hricak, P. Carroll, S.J.

Nelson, and J. Kurhanewicz. "Localization of Prostate Cancer After Hormone Ablation by MRI and 3D 1H MRSI: Case-Control Study with Pathologic Correlation. Presented at Seventh Annual Meeting of the International Society for Magnetic Resonance In Medicine. 3 (1999): 1519.

Byron, P.J., H.E. Butler, A.D. Nelson, and J.P. Lipuma. "Magnetic Resonance Imaging of the Prostate." *American Journal Radiology* 146 (1986): 543–48.

Chen, M., H. Hricak, C.L. Kalbhen, J. Kurhanewicz, D.B. Vigneron, J.M. Weiss, and P.R. Carroll. "Hormonal Ablation of Prostatic Cancer: Effects on Prostate Morphology, Tumor Detection, and Staging by Endorectal Coil Mr Imaging." *American Journal Roentgenol* 166 (1996):1157–63.

Cohen, J.S. "Phospholipid and Energy Metabolism of Cancer Cells Monitored by 31P Magnetic Resonance Spectroscopy: Possible Clinical Significance." *Mayo Clinic Proceedings* 63 (1988): 1199–1207.

Daly, P.F. and J.S. Cohen. "Magnetic Resonance Spectroscopy of Tumors and Potential In Vivo Clinical Applications: A Review." *Cancer Research* 49 (1989): 770–79.

D'Amico, A.V., R. Whittington, S.B. Malkowicz, D. Schultz, M. Schnall, J.E. Tomaszewski, and A. Wein. "Critical Analysis of the Ability of the Endorectal Coil Magnetic Resonance Imaging Scan to Predict Pathologic Stage, Margin Status, and Postoperative Prostate-Specific Antigen Failure in Patients with Clinically Organ-Confined Prostate Cancer." *Journal of Clinical Oncology* 14 (1996): 1770–77.

D'Amico, A.V., R. Whittington, M. Schnall, S.B. Malkowicz, J.E. Tomaszewski, D. Schultz, and A. Wein. "The Impact of the Inclusion of Endorectal Coil Magnetic Resonance Imaging in a Multivariate Analysis to Predict Clinically Unsuspected Extraprostatic Cancer." *Cancer* 75 (1995): 2368–72.

Heerschap, A., G.J. Jager, M. van der Graaf, J.O. Barentsz, J.J. de la Rosette, G.O. Oosterhof, E.T. Ruijter, and S.H. Ruijs. "In Vivo Proton MR 17 Spectroscopy Reveals Altered Metabolite Content in Malignant Prostate Tissue." *Anticancer Research* 17 (1997): 1455–60.

Heerschap, A., G.J. Jager, M. van der Graaf, J.O. Barentsz, and S.H. Ruijs. Proton MR Spectroscopy of the Normal Human

Prostate with an Endorectal Coil and a Double Spin-Echo Pulse Sequence." *Magn Reson Med* 37 (1997): 204–13.

Hricak, H., S. White, D. Vigneron, J. Kurhanewicz, A. Kosco, D. Levin, J. Weiss, P. Narayan and P.R. Carroll. "Carcinoma of the Prostate Gland: MR Imaging With Pelvic Phased-Array Coils Versus Integrated Endorectal—Pelvic Phased-Array Coils, " *Radiology* 193 (1994): 703–9.

Kaji, Y., J. Kurhanewicz, H. Hricak, D. Sokolov, L.R. Huang, S. Nelson, and D. Vigneron. "Localizing Prostate Cancer in the Presence of Postbiopsy Changes On Mr Images: Role of Proton Mr Spectroscopic Imaging." *Radiology* 206 (1998): 785–90.

Kalbhen, C.L., H. Hricak, M. Chen, K. Shinohara, F. Parivar, J. Kurhanewicz, and D. Vigneron. "Prostate Carcinoma: MR Imaging Findings After Cryosurgery." *Radiology* 198 (1996):807–11.

Kurhanewicz, J., R. Dahiya, J.M. MacDonald, L.H. Chang, T.L. James, and P. Narayan. "Citrate Alterations in Primary and Metastatic Human Prostatic Adenocarcinomas: 1H Magnetic Resonance Spectroscopy and Biochemical Study." *Magn Reson Med* 29 (1993): 149–57.

Kurhanewicz, J., D.B. Vigneron, H. Hricak, P. Narayan, P. Carroll, and S.J. Nelson. "Three-Dimensional H-I MR Spectroscopic Imaging of the in Situ Human Prostate with High (O.24-O.7-Cm3) Spatial Resolution." *Radiology* 198 (1996): 795–805.

Kurhanewicz, J., D.B. Vigneron, H. Hricak, F. Parivar, S.J. Nelson, K. Shinohara, and P.R. Carroll. "Prostate Cancer: Metabolic Response to Cryosurgery as Detected with 3D H-I MR Spectroscopic Imaging." *Radiology* 200 (1996):489–96.

Kurhanewicz, J., D.B. Vigneron, and S.J. Nelson, H. Hricak, J.M. MacDonald, B. Konety, and P. Narayan. "Citrate as an In Vivo Marker to Discriminate Prostate Cancer from Benign Prostatic Hyperplasia and Normal Prostate Peripheral Zone: Detection Via Localized Proton Spectroscopy." *Urology* 45 (1995): 459–66.

Liney, G.P., L.W. Turnbull, M. Lowry, L.S. Turnbull, A.J. Knowles, and A. Horsman. "In Vivo Quantification of Citrate Concentration and Water T2 Relaxation Time of the

Pathologic Prostate Gland Using 1H MRS and MRI." *Magnetic Resonance Imaging* 15 (1997):1177–86.

Ling, D., J.K.T. Lee, J.P. Heiken, D.M. Balfe, H.S. Glazer, and G.L. McClennan. "Prostatic Carcinoma and Benign Prostatic Hyperplasia: Inability of MR Imaging to Distinguish Between the Two Diseases." *Radiology* 158 (1986): 103–07.

Lowry, M., G.P. Liney, L.W. Turnbull, D.J. Manton, S.J. Blackband, and A. Horsman. "Quantification of Citrate Concentration in the Prostate by Proton Magnetic Resonance Spectroscopy: Zonal and Age-Related Differences." *Magnetic Resonance in Medicine* 36 (1996):352–58.

Males, R., W. Okuno, D.B. Vigneron, M. Swanson, P. Wood, S.J. Nelson, M. Roach, and J. Kurhanewicz. "Monitoring Effects of Prostate Cancer Brachytherapy Using Combined MRI/MRSI. Presented at Seventh Annual Meeting of the International Society for Magnetic Resonance In Medicine. 1 (1999): 115.

McNeal, J.E., R.A. Kindrachuk, F.S. Freiha, and D.G. Bostwick. A RE, A ST. "Patterns of Progression in Prostate Cancer." *Lancet* 1 (1986): 60–63.

Moyher, S.E., D.B. Vigneron, and S.J. Nelson. "Surface Coil MR Imaging of the Human Brain with an Analytic Reception Profile Correction." *Journal Magn Reson Imaging* 5 (1995): 139–44.

Mueller-Lisse, U.G., J. Kurhanewicz, A. Bessette, R. Males, M. Swanson, A. Fang, S. Nelson, H. Hricak, I. Barken, and D.B. Vigneron. "Hormone Ablation of Localized Prostate Cancer: Effects of Duration of Therapy on Prostate Metabolism Demonstrated by 3D ^{1}H MR Spectroscopy. Presented at Seventh Annual Meeting of the International Society for Magnetic Resonance In Medicine. 3 (1999): 1518.

Parivar, F., H. Hricak, K. Shinohara, J. Kurhanewicz, D.B. Vigneron, S.J. Nelson, and P.R. Carroll. "Detection of Locally Recurrent Prostate Cancer After Cryosurgery: Evaluation by Transrectal Ultrasound, Magnetic Resonance Imaging, and Three-Dimensional Proton Magnetic Resonance Spectroscopy." (1996): 594–99.

Parivar, F. and J. Kurhanewicz. "Detection of Recurrent Prostate Cancer After Cryosurgery." *Current Opinion in Urology* 8 (1998): 83–86.

Partin, A.W., M.W. Kattan, E.N. Subong, P.C. Walsh, K.J. Wojno, J.E. Oesterling, P.T. Scardino, and J.D. Pearson. "Combination of Prostate-Specific Antigen, Clinical Stage, and Gleason Score to Predict Pathological Stage of Localized Prostate Cancer. A Multi-Institutional Update." *Journal of the American Medical Association* 277 (1997):1445–51.

Partin, A.W., J. Yoo, and H.B. Carter et al. "The Use of Prostate Specific Antigen, Clinical Stage and Gleason Score to Predict Pathological Stage in Men with Localized Prostate Cancer." *Journal of Urology* 150 (1993): 110–14.

Partin, A.W., J. Yoo, H.B. Carter, J.D. Pearson, D.W. Chan, J.I. Epstein, and P.C. Walsh. "The Use of Prostate Specific Antigen, Clinical Stage and Gleason Score to Predict Pathological Stage in Men with Localized Prostate Cancer." *Journal of Urology* 150 (1993):110–14.

Phillips, M.E., H.Y. Kressel, C.E. Spritzer, P.H. Arger, A.J. Wein, D. Marinelli, L. Axel, W.B. Gefter, and H.M. Pollack. "Prostatic Disorders: MR Imaging at 1 ST." *Radiology* 164 (1987): 386–92.

Platt J.F., R.L. Bree, and R.E. Schwab. "The Accuracy of CT in the Staging of Carcinoma of the Prostate." *American Journal of Roentgenol* 149 (1987):315–8.

Rifkin, M.D., E.A. Zerhouni, C.A. Gatsonis, L.E. Quint, D.M. Paushter, J.I. Epstein, U. Hamper, P.C. Walsh, B.J. McNeil. "Comparison of Magnetic Resonance Imaging and Ultrasonography in Staging Early Prostate Cancer. Results Of A Multi-Institutional Cooperative Trial." *New England Journal of Medicine* 323 (1990): 621–6.

Scardino, P.T., K. Shinohara, T.M. Wheeler, and S.S Carter. "Staging of Prostate Cancer. Value of Ultrasonography." *Urol Clin North America* 16 (1989):713–34.

Scharen-Guivek, V.L.M., R. Males, S.J. Nelson, U.G. Mueller-Lisse, D.B. Vigneron, and J. Kurhanewicz. "Evaluation of Local Prostate Recurrence after Radical Prostatectomy using Magnetic Resonance Spectrosscopic Imaging." Presented at

Seventh Annual Meeting of the International Society for Magnetic Resonance In Medicine. 1 (1999): 117.

Scheidler, J., H. Hricak, D.B. Vigneron, K.K. Yu, D.L. Sokolov, R.L. Huang, C.J. Zaloudek, S.J. Nelson, P.R. Carroll, and J. Kurhanewicz. "3D 11-I-MR Spectroscopic Imaging in Localizing Prostate Cancer: Clinico-Pathologic Study." *Radiology* (1999 In Press)

Schick, F., H. Bongers, S. Kurz, W.I. Jung, M. Pfeffer, and 0. Lutz. "Localized Proton MR Spectroscopy of Citrate in Vitro and of the Prostate in Vivo at I.5 T." *Magn Reson Med* 29 (1993): 38–43.

Schnall, M.D., Y. Imai, J. Tomaszewski, H.M. Pollack, R.E. Lenkinski, F.Y. Kressel. "Prostate Cancer: Local Staging with Endorectal Surface Coil MR Imaging." *Radiology* 178 (1991): 797–802.

Stamey, T.A. "Cancer of the Prostate: An Analysis of Some Important Contributions and Dilemmas." *Mono Urology* 3 (1982): 67–94.

Victor, T.A., C.A. Lawson, R.C. Wiebolt, S. Nussbaum, M.C. Shattuch, A.G. Brodin, and H. Degani. "Prediction of Hormonal Response of Human Breast Carcinoma by P Spectroscopy." In Hasetine ed. *Magnetic Resonance of the Reproductive System*. New Jersey: Slack, 1987: 67–80.

Vigneron, D., R. Males, H. Hricak, S. Noworolski, P.R. Carrol, and J. Kurhanewicz. "Prostate Cancer: Correlation of 3D MRSI Metabolite Levels with Histologic Grade." Presented at RSNA. 209(P) (1998): 181.

Vigneron, D.B., S.J. Nelson, S. Moyher, D.A.C. Kelley, J. Kurhanewicz, and H. Hricak "An Analytical Correction of MR Images Obtained with Endorectal or Surface Coils. Presented at Society of Magnetic Resonance Imaging Eleventh Annual Meeting. 3(P) (1993): 142.

Vigneron, D., S. Nelson, and J. Surhanewicz. "Proton Chemical Shift Imaging of Cancer." In: Hricak, Higgins and Helms ed. *Magnetic Resonance Imaging of the Body*. New York: Raven Press, 1996: Chapter 12 205–20.

Wice, B.M., G. Trugnan, M. Pinto, M. Rousset, G. Chevalier, E. Dussaulx, B. Lacroix, and A. Zweibaum. "The Intracellular Accumulation Of   UDP=N-Acetylhexosamines

Isconcomitant with the Inability of Human Colon Cancer Cells to Differentiate." *Journal of Biol Chem* 260 (1985): 139–46.

Yu, K.K, J. Scheidler, H. Hricak, D.B. Vigneron, R. Males, C. Zaloudek, S.J. Nelson, P.R. Carroll, and J. Kurhanewicz. "Prostate Cancer: Prediction of

Extracapsular Extension by Endorectal MR Imaging and 3D ^{1}H-MR Spectroscopic Imaging." *Radiology* 1999 (In Press).

Chapter 4 References:

Boyce, W.H. et al. "Ultrasonography as an Aid in the Diagnosis and Management of Surgical Disease of the Pelvis. Special Emphasis on the Genitourinary System." *Ann Surg* 184 (1976): 477.

Chodak, G.W. et al. "Comparison of Digital Examination and Transrectal Ultrasonography for the Diagnosis of Prostate Cancer." *Journal of Urology* 135 (1986): 951.

Cooner, W.H., G.W. Eggers, and P. Lichtenstein. "Prostate Cancer: New Hope for Early Diagnosis." *Ala Med* 56 (1987): 13.

Friedman, A.C. et al. "Relative Merits of MRI, US and CT in the Diagnosis and Staging of Carcinoma of the Prostate." *Urology* 31 (1988): 530.

King, W.W. et al. "Current Status of Prostatic Echography." *JAMA* 266 (1973): 444.

Kudow, C., J.C. Gingell, and J.B. Pinry. "Prostatic Ultrasonography: A Useful Technique?" *Br Journal of Urology* 5 (1985): 440.

Lee, F. et al. "The Use of Transrectal Ultrasound in the Diagnosis, Guided Biopsy, Staging and Screening of Prostate Cancer." *Radiographics* 7 (1987): 627.

Liddell, H.T., W.S. McDougal, D.D. Burks, and A.C. Fleisher. "Ultrasound Versus Digitally Directed Prostate Needle Biopsy." *Journal of Urology* 135 (1986): 716.

Mizuno, S. "Diagnostic Application of Ultrasound in Obstetrics and Gynecology." In C.C. Grossman ed. *Diagnostic Ultrasound*. New York: Plenum Press, 1966: 452.

Resnick, M.I. "Transrectal Ultrasound Guided Versus Digitally Directed Prostatic Biopsy. A Comparative Study." *Journal of Urology* 139 (1988): 754.

Rifkin, M.D., A.B. Kurtz, and B.B. Goldberg. "Sonographically Guided Transperineal Prostate Biopsy: Prelininary Experience with a Longitudinal Linear Airway Transducer." *AJR* 140 (1983): 745.

Rosenberg, S., P.C. Sogani, E.A. Parmer, and D.G. Muller. "Screening of Ambulatory Patients for Prostate Cancer by Transrectal Ultrasonography." *Journal of Urology* 137 (1987): 241A.

Watananbe, H. et al. "Development and Application of New Equipment for Transrectal Ultrasonography." *Journal of Clinical Ultrasound* 2 (1974): 91.

Watananbe, H. et al. "Transrectal Ultrasonography of the Prostate." *Journal of Urology* 114 (1975): 734.

Watananbe, H., H. Kaiho, M. Tanaka, and Y. Terasawa. "Ultrasonographic Diagnosis of the Prostate. II. Sagittal Tomography of the Prostate by Means of B-Mode Scanning." *Medical Ultrason* 9 (1971): 26.

Chapter 5 References:

Amdur, R.J., J.T. Parsons, L.T. Fitzgerald, and R.R. Million. "Adenocarcinoma of the Prostate Treated with External Beam Radiation Therapy: 5-Year Minimum Follow-Up." *Radiother Oncology* 19(3) (1990): 235–46.

Anscher, M.S. and L.R. Prosnitz. "Radiotherapy Vs. Hormonal Therapy for the Management of Locally Recurrent Prostate Cancer Following Radical Prostatectomy." *Int J Radiat Oncology Biol Phys* 5(17) (1989): 953–58.

Aristizabal, S.A., D. Steinbronn, and R.S. Heusinkveld. "External Beam Radiotherapy In Cancer of the Prostate." *Radiother Oncology* 1 (1984): 309–15.

Austin-Seymour, M., R. Caplan, and K. Russell et al. "Impact of a Multileaf Collimator on Treatment M Orbidity in Localized Carcinoma of the Prostate." *Int J Radiat Oncol Biol Phys* 30(5) (1994): 1065–71.

Bagshaw, M.A., R.S. Cox, and G.R. Ray. "Status of Radiation Treatment of Prostate Cancer at Stamford University." In: *Consensus Development Conference on the Management of Clinically Localized Prostate Cancer. National Cancer Institute Monographs.* No. 7. Washington, D.C.: Government Printing Office, 1988: 47–60.

Bahnson, R.R., J.E. Garnett, and J.T. Grayhack. "Adjuvant Radiation Therapy in Stage C And D, Prostatic Adenocarcinoma: Preliminary Results." *Urology* 27(5) (1986): 403–06.

Bolla, M., D. Gonzalez, and P. Warde et al. "Immediate Hormonal Therapy Improves Locoregional Control and Survival in Patients with Locally Advanced Prostate Cancer. Results of a Randomized Phase III Clinical Trial of the EORTC Radiotherapy and Genito-Urinary Tract Cancer Cooperative Groups." *Proceedings of American Soc Clinical Oncology* 15 (1996): 238.

Boring, C.C., T.S. Squires, and T. Tong. "Cancer Statistics" 1993. Ca 4 3(1) (1993): 7–26.

Brock, W.A., S.L. Tucker, and F.B. Geara et al. "Fibroblast Radiosensitivity Versus Acute and Late Normal Skin Responses in Patients Treated for Breast Cancer." *Int J Radiat Oncol Biol Phys* 32 (1995): 1371–79.

Burnet, N.G., J. Nyman, and I. Turesson et al. "The Relationship Between Cellular Radiation Sensitivity and Tissue Response May Provide the Basis for Individualizing Radiotherapy Schedules." *Radiother Oncology* 33 (1994): 228–38.

Cancer Research Campaign. Cancer of the prostate. Factsheet 20(1), 1994.

Carter, G.E., G. Lieskovsky, D.G. Skinner, and Z. Petrovich. "Results of Local and/or Systemic Adjuvant Therapy in the Management of Pathological Stage C or D1 Prostate Cancer Following Radical Prostatectomy." *Journal of Urology* 142 (1989): 1266–71.

Cheng, W.S., M. Frydenberg, and E.J. Bergstralh et al. "Radical Prostatectomy for Pathologic Stage C Prostate Cancer: Influence of Pathologic Variables and Adjuvant Treatment on Disease Outcome." *Urology* 42(3) (1993): 283–91.

Chodak, G.W., R.A. Thisted, and G.S. Gerber et al. "Results of Conservative Management of Clinically Localized Prostate

Cancer." *New England Journal of Medicine* 330(4) (1994): 242–48.

Critz, F.A., A.K. Levinson, W.J. Williams, and D.A. Holladay. "Prostate-Specific Antigen Nadir: The Optimum Level After Irradiation for Prostate Cancer." *Journal of Clinical Oncology* 14(11) (1996): 2893–00.

Crook, J., S. Robertson, and G. Collin et al. "Clinical Relevance of Trans-Rectal Ultrasound, Biopsy and Serum Prostate-Specific Antigen Following External Beam Radiotherapy for Carcinoma of the Prostate." Int J Radiat Oncol Biol Phys 27(1) (1993): 31–37.

Dattoli, M., K. Wallner, and R. Sorace et al. "103Pd Brachytherapy and External Beam Irradiation for Clinically Localized, High-Risk Prostatic Carcinoma." *Int J Radiat Oncol Biol Phys* 35(5) (1996): 875–79.

Dearnaley, D.P. "Radiotherapy for Prostate Cancer: The Changing Scene." *Clinical Oncology* 7(2) (1995): 147–50.

Dearnaley, D.P. "Radiotherapy of Prostate Cancer: Established Results and New Developments." *Semin Surg Oncol* 11(1) (1995): 50–59.

Dearnaley, D.P., A. Horwich, and R.J. Shearer. "Treatment of Advanced Localized Prostatic Cancer by Orchiectomy, Radiotherapy or Combined Treatment. A Medical Research Council Study." *Br Journal of Urology* 72(5[I]) (1992): 673–74.

Dearnaley, D.P., A. Nahum, and M. Lee et al. "Radiotherapy of Prostate Cancer. Reducing the Treated Volume. Conformal Therapy, Hormone Cytoreduction and Protons." *Br Journal of Cancer* 70(suppl 22) (1994): 16.

Dearnaley, D.P., R.J. Shearer, and L. Ellingham et al. "Rationale and Initial Results of Adjuvant Hormone Therapy and Irradiation for Localized Prostate Cancer." In: M. Motta and M. Serio eds. *Sex Hormone and Antihormones in Endocrine Dependent Pathology: Basic and Clinical Aspects*. Amsterdam: Elsevier Science, 1994: 197–08.

de Jong, B., M. Crommelin, L.H. van der Heijden, and J.W.W. Coebergh. "Patterns of Radiotherapy for Cancer Patients in South-Eastern Netherlands, 1975–1989." *Radiother Oncology* 31 (1994): 213–21.

DeWit, L., K.K. Ang, and E. van der Schueren. "Acute Side Effects and Late Complications After Radiotherapy of Localized Carcinoma of the Prostate." *Cancer Treatment Review* 10 (1983): 79–89.

Duncan, W., P. Warde, and C.N. Catton et al. "Carcinoma of the Prostate: Results of Radica L Radiotherapy (1970–1985)." *Int J Radiat Oncol Biol Phys* 26(2) (1993): 203–10.

Dusserre, A., G. Garavaglia, J.Y. Giraud, and M. Bolla. "Quality Assurance of the EORTC Radiotherapy Trial 22863 for Prostatic Cancer: The Dummy Run." *Radiother Oncology* 36 (1995): 229–34.

Early Breast Cancer Trialists' Collaborative Group. "Systemic Treatment of Early Breast Cancer by Hormonal, Cytotoxic, or Immune Therapy (Part I)." *Lancet* 339(8784) (1992): 1–15.

Early Breast Cancer Trialists' Collaborative Group. "Systemic Treatment of Early Breast Cancer by Hormonal, Cytotoxic, or Immune Therapy (Part II)." *Lancet* 339(8785) (1992): 71–85.

Effleston, J.C. and P.C. Walsh. "Radical Prostatectomy with Preservation of Sexual Function: Pathological Findings in the First 100 Cases." *Journal of Urology* 134(6) (1985): 1146–48.

Eisburch, A., C.A. Perez, E.H. Roessler, and M.A. Lockett. "Adjuvant Irradiation After Prostatectomy for Carcinoma of the Prostate with Positive Surgical Margins." *Cancer* 73(2) (1994): 384–87.

Emami, B., J. Lyman, and A. Brown et al. "Tolerance of Normal Tissue to Therapeutic Radiation." *Int J Radiat Oncol Biol Phys* 21 (1991): 109–22.

Epstein, B.E. and G.E. Hanks. "Radiation Therapy Techniques and Dose Selection in the Treatment Of Prostate Cancer." *Semin Radiat Oncology* 3(3) (1993): 179–86.

Fellows, G.J., P.B. Clark, and L.L. Beynon et al. "Treatment of Advanced Localized Prostatic Cancer by Orchiectomy, Radiotherapy, or Combined Treatment: A Medical Research Council Study." *Br Journal of Urology* 70 (1992): 304–09.

Feneley, M.R., D.A. Gillatt, M. Hehir, and R.S. Kirby. "A Review of Radical Prostatectomy from Three Centers in the UK:

Clinical Presentation and Outcome." *Br Journal of Urology* 78(6) (1996): 911–20.

Forman, J.D., E. Zinreich, and L. Ding-Jen et al. "Improving the Therapeutic Ratio of External Beam Irradiation for Carcinoma of the Prostate." *Int J Radiat Oncol Biol Phys* 11 (1985): 2073–80.

Fransson, P., A. Widmark. "Self-Assessed Sexual Function After Pelvic Irradiation for Prostate Carcinoma. Comparison with an Age-Matched Control Group." *Cancer* 78(5) (1996): 1066–78.

Freeman, J.A., G. Lieskovsky, and D.W. Cook et al. "Radical Retropubic Prostatectomy and Post-Operative Adjuvant Radiation for Pathological Stage C(Pcn$_0$) Prostate Cancer From 1976 To 1989: Intermediate Findings." *Journal of Urology* 149(5) (1993): 1029–34.

Freiha, F.S. and M.A. Bagshaw. "Carcinoma of the Prostate: Results of Post-Irradiation Biopsy." *Prostate* 5(1) (1984): 19–25.

Fuks, Z., S.A. Leibel, and K.E. Wallner et al. "The Effect of Local Control on Metastatic Dissemination in Carcinoma of the Prostate: Long Term Results in Patients Treated with I Implantation." *Int J Radiat Oncol Biol Phys* 21(3) (1991): 537–47.

Goffinet, D.R. and M.A. Baghaw. "Radiation Therapy of Prostate Carcinoma: Thirty-Year Experience at Stanford University." In: F.H. Schroder, ed. *EORTC Genitourinary Group Monograph 8. Treatment of Prostatic Cancer—Facts and Controversies*. New York: Wiley-Liss Inc., 1990: 209–22.

Griffin, D.T.W. "Fast Neutron Irradiation Of Locally Advanced Prostate Cancer." *Semin Oncology* 15(4) (1988): 359.

Hanks, G.E. "Treatment of Early Stage Prostate Cancer: Radiotherapy." In: V.T. DeVita, S. Hellman, and S.A. Rosenberg, eds. *Important Advances in Oncology*. Philadelphia: J.B. Lippincott, 1994: 225–39.

Hanks, G.E., S. Asbell, and J.M. Krall et al. "Outcome for Lymph Node Dissection Negative T-1b, T-2 (A-2,B) Prostate Cancer Treated with External Beam Radiation Therapy In RTOG 77-06." Int J Radiat Oncol Biol Phys 21(4) (1991): 1099–03.

Hanks, G.E., B.W. Corn, W.R. Lee, M. Hunt, A. Hanlon, and T.E. Schultheiss. "External Beam Irradiation Of Prostate Cancer: Conformal Treatment Techniques and Outcomes for the 1990s." *Cancer* 75 (1995): 1972–77.

Hanks, G.E. and A.K. Dawson "The Role of External Beam Radiation Therapy After Prostatectomy for Prostate Cancer." *Cancer* 58 (1986): 2406–10.

Hanks, G.E., J.J. Diamond, and J.M. Krall et al. "A Ten Year Follow-Up of 682 Patients Treated F or Prostate Cancer with Radiation Therapy in the United States." *Int J Radiat Oncol Biol Phys* 13(4) (1987): 499–05.

Hanks, G.E., A.L. Hanlon, and G. Hudes et al. "Patterns-of-Failure Analysis of Patients with High Pretreatment Prostate-Specific Antigen Levels Treated by Radiation Therapy: The Need for Improved Systemic and Locoregional Treatment." *Journal Clinical Oncology* 14(4) (1996): 1093–97.

Hanks, G.E., A. Hanlon, J.B. Owen, and T.E. Schultheiss. "Patterns of Radiation Treatment of Elderly Patients with Prostate Cancer." *Cancer* 74(suppl 7) (1994): 2174–77.

Hanks, G.E., J.M. Krail, and K.L. Martz et al. "The Outcome of Treatment of 313 Patients with T1 (UICC) Prostate Cancer Treated with External Beam Irradiation." *Int J Radiat Oncol Biol Phys* 14(2) (1988): 243–48.

Hanks, G.E., W.R. Lee, and A.L. Hanlon et al. "Conformal Technique Dose Escalation for Prostate Cancer: Biochemical Evidence of Improved Cancer Control with Higher Doses in Patients with Pretreatment Prostate-Specific Antigen." >10 ng/ml. *Int J Radiat Oncol Biol Phys* 35(5) (1996): 861–68.

Hanks, G.E., K.L. Martz, and J.J. Diamond. "The Effect of Dose on Local Control of Prostate Cancer." *Int J Radiat Oncol Biol Phys* 15(6) (1988): 1299–05.

Hartford, A.C., A. Niemierko, and J.A. Adams et al. "Conformal Irradiation of the Prostate: Estimating Long-Term Rectal Bleeding Risk Using Dose-Volume Histograms." *Int J Radiat Oncol Biol Phys* 36(3) (1996): 721–30.

Helgason, A.R., M. Fredrikson, J. Adolfsson, and G. Steineck. "Decreased Sexual Capacity After External Radiation Therapy for Prostate Cancer Impairs Quality of Life." *Int J Radiat Oncol Biol Phys* 32(1) (1995): 33–39.

Horwitz, E.M., F.A. Vicini, and E.L. Ziaja et al. "Assessing the Variability of Outcome for Patients Treated with Localized Prostate Irradiation Using Different Definitions of Biochemical Control." *Int J Radiat Oncol Biol Phys* 36(3) (1996): 565–71.

ICRU report 29. Dose specification for reporting external beam therapy with photons and electrons. Washington, D.C.: International Commission on Radiation Units and Measurements, April 1, 1978.

Johansen, J., S.M. Bentzen, J. Overgaard, and M. Overgaard. "Relationship Between the In Vitro Radiosensitivity of Skin Fibroblasts and the Expression of Subcutaneous Fibrosis, Telangiectasia, and Skin Erythema After Radiotherapy." *Radiother Oncology* 40(2) (1996): 101–09.

Kaplan, E.L. and P. Meier. "Nonparametric Estimation from Incomplete Observations." *Journal American Stat Association* 53 (1958): 457–81.

Kutcher, G.J. and C. Burman. "Calculation of Complication Probability Factors for Non-Uniform Normal Tissue Irradiation: The Effective Volume Method." *Int J Radiat Oncol Biol Phys* 16(6) (1989): 1623–30.

Kutcher, G.J., C. Burman, and L. Brewster et al. "Histogram Reduction Method for Calculating Complication Probabilities for Three-Dimensional Treatment Planning Evaluations." *Int J Radiat Oncol Biol Phys* 21 (1991): 137–46.

Lange, P.H., D.J. Lightner, and E. Medini et al. "The effect of Radiation Therapy After Radical Prostatectomy in Patients with Elevated Prostate Specific Antigen Levels." *Journal of Urology* 144(4) (1990): 927–33.

Lange, P.H., T.D. Moon, P. Narayan, and E. Medini. "Radiation Therapy as Adjuvant Treatment After Radical Prostatectomy: Patient Tolerance and Preliminary Results." *Journal of Urology* 136 (1986): 45–49.

Lange, P.H. and P. Narayan. "Understaging and Undergrading of Prostate Cancer. Argument for Postoperative Radiation as Adjuvant Therapy." *Urology* 21(2) (1983): 113–18.

Lee, M., C. Wynne, and S. Webb et al. "A Comparison of Proton And Megavoltage X-Ray Treatment Planning for Prostate Cancer." *Radiother Oncology* 33(3) 1994: 239–53.

Leibel, S.A., Z. Fuks, M.J. Zelefsky, and W.F. Whitmore Jr. "The Effects of Local and Regional Treatment on the Metastatic Outcome in Prostatic Carcinoma with Pelvic Lymph Node Involvement." *Int J Radiat Oncol Biol Phys* 28 (1994): 7–16.

Leibel, S.A., G.E. Hanks, and S. Kramer. "Patterns of Care Outcome Studies: Results of the National Practice in Adenocarcinoma of the Prostate." *Int J Radiat Oncol Biol Phys* 10(3) (1984): 401–09.

Leibel S.A., R. Heimann, and G.J. Kutcher et al. "Three-Dimensional Conformal Radiation Therapy in Locally Advanced Carcinoma of the Prostate: Preliminary Results of a Phase I Dose-Escalation Study." *Int J Radiat Oncol Biol Phys* 28(1) (1994): 55–65.

Leibel, S.A., M.J. Zelefsky, and G.J. Kutcher et al. "The Biological Basis and Clinical Application of Three-Dimensional Conformal External Beam Radiation Therapy in Carcinoma of the Prostate." *Semin Oncology* 21(5) (1994): 580–97.

Lu-Yao, G.L., D. McLerran, J. Wasson, and J.E. Wannber. "An Assessment of Radical Prostatectomy. Time Trends, Geographic Variation, and Outcomes. The Prostate Patient Outcomes Research Team." *JAMA* 269 (1993): 2633–36.

Lyman, J.T. "Complication Probability as Assessed from Dose-Volume Histograms." *Radiat Research* 22 (1985): 355–59.

McLaughlin, P.W., H.M. Sandler, M.R. Jiroutek. "Prostate-specific antigen following prostate radiotherapy: how low can you go?" *Journal of Clinical Oncology* 14(11) 1996: 2889–92.

McNeil, C. "PSA Levels After Radiotherapy: How Low Must They Go?" *Journal National Cancer Institute* 88(12) (1996): 791–92.

Mentel, N. "Evaluation of Survival Data and Two New Rank Order Statistics Arising in its Consideration." *Cancer Chemotherapy Report* 50 (1966): 163–70.

Mesina, C.F., R. Sharman, and L.S. Rissman et al. "Comparison of a Standard Four-Field Boost Technique with a Customized Non-Axial External Beam Technique for the Treatment of Adenocarcinoma of the Prostate." *Int J Radiat Oncol Biol Phys* 27(suppl 1) (1993): 193.

Mettlin, C. "The Status of Prostate Cancer Early Detection." *Cancer* 72 (supplement 3) 1993: 1050–55.

Mithal, N.P. and P.J. Hoskin. "External Beam Radiotherapy for Carcinoma of the Prostate: A Retrospective Study." *Clinical Oncology* 5(5) (1993): 297–01.

Munro, A.J. "An Overview of Randomized Controlled Trial of Adjuvant Chemotherapy in Head and Neck Cancer." *Br Journal of Cancer* 71(1) (1995): 83–91.

Nahum, A.E., D.P. Dearnaley, and G.G. Steel. "Prospects for Proton-Beam Radiotherapy." *European Journal of Cancer* 30A(10) (1994): 1577–83.

National Institutes of Health Consensus Development Panel. Consensus statement: the management of clinically localized prostate cancer. In: Consensus Development Conference on the Management of Clinically Localized Prostate Cancer. National Cancer Institute monographs. No. 7. Washington, D.C.: Government Printing Office, 1988: 3–6.

Neal, A.J., M. Oldham, and D.P. Dearnaley. "Comparison of Treatment Techniques for Conformal Radiotherapy of the Prostate Using Dose-Volume Histograms and Normal Tissue Complication Probabilities." *Radiother Oncology* 37(1) (1995): 29–34.

Neglia, W.J., D.H. Hussey, and D.E. Johnson. "Megavoltage Radiation Therapy for Carcinoma of the Prostate." *Int J Radiat Oncol Biol Phys* 2 (1977): 873–83.

Pelipich, M.V., J.M. Krall, and M. al-Saffaf et al. "Androgen Deprivation with Radiation Therapy Compared with Radiation Therapy Alone for Locally Advanced Prostatic Carcinoma: A Randomized Comparative Trial of the Radiation Therapy Oncology Group." *Urology* 45 (1995): 616–23.

Perez, C.A., M.V. Pilepich, and D. Garcia et al. "Definitive Radiation Therapy in Carcinoma of the Prostate Localized to the Pelvis: Experience at the Mallinckrodt Institute of Radiology. *NCI Monogr* 7 (1988): 85–94.

Perez, C.A., B.J. Walz, and F.R. Zivnuska. "Irradiation of Carcinoma of the Prostate Localized to the Pelvis: Analysis of Tumor Response and Prognosis." *Int J Radiat Oncol Biol Phys* 6(5) (1980): 555–63.

Pilepich, M.V., S.O. Asbell, and J.M. Krall et al. "Correlation of Radiotherapeutic Parameters and Treatment Related Morbidity—Analysis of RTOG Study 77–06." *Int J Radiat Oncol Biol Phys* 13(7) (1987): 1007–12.

Pilepich, M.V., R. Caplan, and R.W. Byhardt et al. "Phase III of Androgen Suppression Using Goserelin in Unfavorable Prognosis Carcinoma of the Prostate Treated with Definitive Radiotherapy (Report of RTOG Protocol 85–31)." *Proceedings American Soc Clinical Oncology* 14 (1995): 239.

Pilepich, M.V., J.M. Krall, and M. al-Sarraf et al. "Androgen Deprivation with Radiation Therapy Compared with Radiation Therapy Alone for Locally Advanced Prostatic Carcinoma: A Randomized Comparative Trial of RTOG." *Urology* 45 (1995): 616–23.

Pilepich, M.V., J.M. Krall, and W.T. Sause et al. "Prognostic Factors in Carcinoma of the Prostate—Analysis of RTOG Study 7506." *Int J Radiat Oncol Biol Phys* 13(3) (1987): 339–49.

Pocock, S.J. and R. Simon. "Sequential Treatment Assignment with Balancing for Prognostic Factors in the Controlled Clinical Trial." *Biometrics* 31 (1975): 103–15.

Powles, T.J., T.F. Hickish, and A. Makris et al. "Randomized Trial of Chemoendocrine Therapy Started Before or After Surgery for Treatment of Primary Breast Cancer." *Journal of Clinical Oncology* 13(3) (1995): 547–52.

Ray, G.R., M.A. Bagshaw, and F. Freiha. "External Beam Radiation Salvage for Residual or Recurrent Local Tumor Following Radical Prostatectomy." *Journal of Urology* 132(5) (1984): 926–30.

Roach, M.I., D.M. Chinn, J. Holland, and M. Clarke. "A Pilot Survey of Sexual Function and Quality of Life Following 3D Conformal Radiotherapy for Clinically Localized Prostate Cancer." *Int J Radiat Oncol Biol Phys* 35(5) (1996): 869–74.

Rosenthal S.A., M. Roach III, and B.J. Goldsmith et al. "Immobilization Improved the Reproducibility of Patient Positioning During Six-Field Conformal Radiation Therapy for Prostate Carcinoma." *Int J Radiat Oncol Biol Phys* 27(4) (1993): 921–26.

Rozan, R., E. Albuisson, and B. Kin et al. "External Beam Radiation of Stage T3/T4 Adenocarcinoma of the Prostate." In:

M. Bolla, J.J. Rambeaud, and F. Vincent eds. *Local Prostatic Carcinoma*. Basel, Switzerland: Karger, 1994: 98–110.

Russell, K.J. "Current Research Directions in the Radiation Therapy of Localized Prostate Cancer." In: N.A. Dawson and N.J. Vogelzang, eds. *Prostate Cancer*. New York: Wiley, 1994: 133–49.

Russell, K.J. and J.C. Blasko. "Recent Advances in Interstitial Brachytherapy for Localized Prostate Cancer." In: P.H. Lange and D.F. Paulson eds. *Problems in Urology: Therapeutic Strategies in Prostate Cancer*. Hagerstown, MD: Lippincott, 7 (1993): 260–79.

Russell, K.J., R.J. Caplan, and G.E. Laramore et al. "Photon Versus Fast Neutron External Beam Radiotherapy in the Treatment of Locally Advanced Prostate Cancer: Results of a Randomized Prospective Trial." *Int J Radiat Oncol Biol Phys* 28(1) (1994): 47–54.

Sagerman, R.H., H.C. Chun, and G.A. King et al. "External Beam Radiotherapy for Carcinoma of the Prostate." *Cancer* 63(12) (1989): 2468–74.

Sailer, S.L., J.G. Rosenman, and J.R. Symon et al. "The Tetrad and Hexad: Maximum Beam Separation as a Starting Point for Noncoplanar 3-D Treatment Planning: Prostate Cancer as a Test Case." *Int J Radiat Oncol Biol Phys* 30(2) (1994): 439–46.

Sandler, H., P.W. McLaughlin, and R. Ten Haken et al. "3D Conformal Radiotherapy for the Treatment of Prostate Cancer: Low Risk of Chronic Rectal Morbidity Observed In a Large Series of Patients." *Int J Radiat Oncol Biol Phys* 27(suppl 1) (1993): 135.

Sandler, H.M., C. Perez-Tomayo, R.K. Ten Haken, and A.S.Lichter. "Dose Escalation for Stage C (T3) Prostate Cancer: Minimal Rectal Toxicity Observed Using Conformal Therapy." *Radiother Oncology* 23(1) (1992): 53–54.

Sause, W.T., C. Scott, and S. Taylor et al. "Radiation Therapy Oncology Group (RTOG) 88–08 and Eastern Cooperative Oncology Group (ECOG) 4588: Preliminary Results of a Phase III Trial in Regionally Advanced, Unresectable Non-Small-Cell Lung Cancer." *Journal of National Cancer Institute* 87(3) (1995): 198–05.

Scardino, P.T. and F. Bretas. "Interstitial Radiotherapy." In: A.W. Bruce and J. Trachtenberg, eds. *Adenocarcinoma of the Prostate*. London: Springer-Verlag, 1987: 145–58.

Scardino, P.T. and T.M. Wheeler. "Local Control of Prostate Cancer with Radiotherapy: Frequency and Prognostic Significance of Positive Results of Postirradiation Prostate Biopsy." In: *Consensus Development Conference on the Management of Clinically Localized Prostate Cancer. National Cancer Institute monographs*. No. 7. Washington, D.C.: Government Printing Office, 1988: 95–103.

Schild, S.E. "Regarding Prost-Operative Radiotherapy for Pathologic Stage C Prostate Cancer: In Response to Dr. Lawrence and Mr. Collins." *Int J Radiat Oncol Biol Phys* 36(3) (1996): 757–59.

Schild, S.E., S.J. Buskirk, and W.W. Wong et al. "The Use of Radiotherapy for Patients with Isolated Elevation of Serum Prostate Specific Antigen Following Radical Prostatectomy." *Journal of Urology* 156(5) (1996): 1725–29.

Schild, S.E., W.W. Wong, and G.L. Grado et al. "The Results of Radical Retropubic Prostatectomy and Adjuvant Therapy for Pathological Stage C Prostate Cancer." *Int J Radiat Oncol Biol Phys* 34(3) (1996): 535–41.

Schroder, F.H. "Screening for Prostate Cancer (letter)." *Lancet* 343(8910) (1994): 1438–39.

Schroder, F.H. "What is New in Endocrine Therapy of Prostatic Cancer?" In: D.W.W. Newling and W.G. Jones eds. *EORTC Genitourinary Group Monograph 7. Prostate Cancer and Testicular Cancer*. New York: Wiley-Liss, 1990: 45–52.

Shearer, R.J., J.H. Davies, J.S.K. Gelister, and D.P. Dearnaley. "Hormonal Cytoreduction and Radiotherapy for Carcinoma of the Prostate." *Br Journal of Urology* 69(5) 1992: 521–24.

Shipley, W.U., L.J. Verhey, and J.E. Munzenrider et al. "Advanced Prostate Cancer: The Results of a Randomized Comparative Trial of High Dose Irradiation Boosting with Conformal Protons Compared with Conventional Dose Irradiation Using Photons Alone." *Int J Radiat Oncol Biol Phys* 32(1) (1995): 3–12.

Steel, G.G. "Combined Radiotherapy-Chemotherapy: Principles." In: G.G. Steel, G.E. Adams, and A. Horwich, eds. *The Biological Basis of Radiotherapy*, 2ⁿᵈ edn. Oxford: Elsevier Science, (1989): 267–89.

Taylor, W.J., R.G. Richardson, and M.D. Hafermann. "Radiation Therapy for Localized Prostate Cancer." *Cancer* 43 (1979): 1123–27.

Ten Haken R.K., C. Perez-Tamayo, and R.J. Tesser et al. "Boost Treatment of the Prostate Using Shaped, Fixed Fields." *Int J Radiat Oncol Biol Phys* 16(1) (1989): 193–00.

Van der Werf-Messing, B., V. Sourek-Zikova, and D.I. Blonk. "Localized Advanced Carcinoma of the Prostate: Radiation Therapy Versus Hormonal Therapy." *Int J Radiat Oncol Biol Phys* 1 (1976): 1043–4 8.

Wallner, K.E. "Iodine Brachytherapy for Early Stage Prostate Cancer. New Techniques May Achieve Better Results." *Oncology* 5 1991: 115–22.

Wallner, K.E., J. Roy, and L. Harrison. "Tumor Control and Morbidity Following Transperineal Iodine Implantation for Stage T1/T2 Prostatic Carcinoma." *Int J Radiat Oncol Biol Phys* 14(2) (1996): 449–53.

Webb, S. and A.E. Nahum. "A model for Calculating Tumor Control Probability in Radiotherapy Including the Effects of Inhomogeneous Distribution of Dose and Clonogenic Cell Density." *Phys Med Biol* 38 (1993): 653–66.

WHO handbook for reporting results of cancer treatment. Geneva: World Health Organization, 1979.

Yorke, E.D., Z. Fuks, and L. Norton et al. "Modeling the Development of Metastases From Primary and Locally Recurrent Tumors: Comparison With a Clinical Data Base for Prostatic Cancer." *Cancer Research* 53 (1993): 2987–93.

Zagars, G.K., A.C. von Eschenbach, D.E. Johnson, and J.M. Oswald. "The Role of Radiation Therapy in Stages A2 and B Adenocarcinoma of the Prostate. *Int J Radiat Oncol Biol Phys* 14 (1988): 701–09.

Zagars, G.K., A.C. von Eschenback, D.E. Johnson, and M.J. Oswald. "Stage C Adenocarcinoma of the Prostate: An Anal-

ysis of 551 Patients Treated with External Beam Radiation."
Cancer 60(7) (1987): 1489–99.

Zietman, A.L., W.U. Shipley, and G.C. Willett. "Residual Disease After Radical Surgery or Radiation Therapy for Prostate Cancer. Clinical Significance and Therapeutic Implications." *Cancer* 71 (1993): 859–69.

Zietman, A.L., M.K. Tibbs, and K.C. Dallow et al. "Use of PSA Nadir to Predict Subsequent Biochemical Outcome Following External Beam Radiation Therapy for T1-2 Adenocarcinoma of the Prostate." *Radiother Oncol* 40(2) (1996): 159–62.

Chapter 6 References:

Dendrathema (Chrysanthemum) Morifolium Tzvel: He et al., *Journal of Natural Products*, 1994, 57(1), pp.42–51.

Ganoderma lucidum Karst: Maruyama et al., J. Pharmacobiodyn, 1989(2), pp.118–23.

Ganoderma lucidum Karst, ed. New Medical College of Jian-Su Province, *Encyclopedia of Chinese Medicinal Herbs*, Shanghai People's Pushisher, 1975, pp. 2395–99.

Glcyrrhiza glabra L.: Kobayashis et al., Bio Pharm Bull, (1995)(10). pp. 1382–85.

Haicka, H. Dorota et al. "Apoptosis and Cell Cycle Effects Induced by Extracts of the Chinese Herbal Preparation PC SPES." *International Journal of Oncology*, Vol. 11 (1997).

Hsieh, Tze-chen et al. "Regulation of Androgen Receptor (AR) and Prostate Specific Antigen (PSA) Expression in the Androgen-Responsive Human Prostate Lncap Cells by Ethanolic Extracts of the Chinese Herbal Preparation, PC SPES." *Biochemistry and Molecular Biology International* Vol. 42, No. 3 (1997): 535–44.

Isatis Indigotica Fort: Xu et al., Chun-His-I-Chieh-Ho-Tsa-Chin, 1991(6). pp. 357–59, 3225–26.

Li ot oi, Cell Molecular Biology Research, (1993): 39(22), 3225–26.

Rubdosia rubescens: Wang et al., Chung Hun-Chung-Liu-Tsa-Chih, 1996(4): 297–99.

Scutellaria baicalensis Georgi: Butenko et al., Agents Actions, Special No. 39, 1993: pp. 49–51.

Scutelleria baiculensis Georgi: Konoshitna et al., Chem Pharm Bull, Tokyo, 1992(2): pp.5 31–33.

Scutelleria baicalensis Georgi: nagai et al., Biol Pharm Bull, 1995(2): pp. 285–89.

Serenca repens: Dralkorn et al., Urologe A., 1995: 34(2) pp. 119–29.

Chapter 7 References:

Critz, F.A., A.K. Levinson, W.H. Williams, D.A. Holladay, and C.T. Holladay. "The PSA Nadir that Indicated Potential Cure After Radiotherapy for Prostate Cancer." *Urology* 49:3 (March 1997): 322–26.

Critz, F.A., A.K. Levinson, W.H. Williams, D.A. Holladay, C.T. Holladay and V.D. Griffin. "Prostate Nadir of 0.5 ng/ml or Less Defines Disease Freedom for Surgically Staged Men Irradiated for Prostate Cancer." *Urology* 49 (1997): 668–672.

Critz, F.A., A.K. Levinson, W.H. Williams, D.A. Holladay, C.T. Holladay and V.D. Griffin. "The PSA Nadir Goal for Radiotherapy of Prostate Cancer is .2. ng/ml." *Urology* 159, Suppl. #5 (1998): 218.

Critz, F.A., A.K. Levinson, W.H. Williams, D.A. Holladay, C.T. Holladay and V.D. Griffin. "Simultaneous Radiotherapy for Prostate Cancer: Prostate Implant Followed by External Beam Radiation." *The Cancer Journal from Scientific American* Vol. 4, No. 6 (November/December 1998).

D'Amico, A.V., R. Whittington, S.B. Malkowicz, D. Schultz, and K. Blank. "Biochemical Outcome After Radical Prostatectomy, External Beam Radiation Therapy, or Interstitial Radiation Therapy for Clinically Localized Prostate Cancer." *Journal of the American Medical Association 280* #11 (1998): 969–974.

Lu-Yau, G.L., A.L. Potosky, P.C. Albertsen, J.H. Wasson, M.J. Barry, and J.E. Wennberg. "Follow-up Prostate Cancer Treatments After Radical Prostatectomy: A Population-Based Study." *Journal of the National Cancer Institute* Vol. 88 No. ®, (February 21, 1998): 166–173.

Stock, R.G., N.N. Stone, J.K. DeWyngaert, P. Lavagnini, and P.D. Unger. "Prostate Specific Antigen Findings and Biopsy Results Following Interactive Ultrasound Guided Transperineal Brachytherapy for Early Stage Prostate Carcinoma." *Cancer* 77 (11) (1996): 2386–92.

Chapter 8 References:

Eary, J.F., C. Collins, M. Stabin, et. al. "Samarium-153-EDTMP Biodistribution and Acsimetry Estimation." *Journal Nucl. Medicine* 34 (1993): 1031–1036.

Farhangi, M., R.A. Holmes, W.A. Volkert, K.W. Logan, and A. Singh. "Samarium-153-EDTMP: Parmacokinetic, toxicity and pain response using an escalating dose schedule in the treatment of metastatic bone cancer. *Journal Nucl. Medicine* 33 (1992): 1451–1458.

Bayouth, J.E., D.E. Macey, L.P. Kasi, and F.V. Fossella. "Dosimetry and toxicity of samarium-153-EDTMP Administered for Bone Pain Due to Skeletal Metastases." *Journal Nucl. Medicine* 35 (1994): 63–69.

Goeckeler, W.F., L.K. Stoneburner, L.P. Kasi et al. "Analysis of Urine Samples from Metastatic Bone Cancer Patients Administered 153Sm-EDTMP." *Nucl. Med. Biol.* 20, 5 (1993): 657–661

Resche, I. J.F. Chatal, A. Pecking et al. *A Dose-controlled Study of 153Sm-Ethylenediaminetetramethylenephosphonate (EDTMP) in the Treatment of Patients with Painful Bone Metastases." Eur. Journal of Cancer* 14, 10 (1997): 1583–91.

Serafini, A.N., S.J. Houston, I. Resche et al. "Palliation of Pain Associated with Mestastatic Bone Cancer Using Samarium SM 153 Lexidronam: A Double Blind Placebo-Controlled Trial." *Journal of Clinical Oncology* 16, 4, (1998): 1574–81.

Chapter 9 References:

Amato, R.J., C.J. Logothetis, F.H. Dexus, A. Sella, R.G. Kilbourn, and K. Fitz. "Preliminary Results of a Phase II Trial of Estramustine (EMCYT) and Vinblastine (VLB) for Patients with Progressive Hormone-Refractory Prostate Carcinoma

(HPRC)." *Proceedings of American Association of Cancer Research* (1991): 32, 86 (abstr. 1111).

Eisenberger, M.A., L.M. Reyno, and D.I. Jodrell et al. "Suramin, an Active Drug for Prostate Cancer: Interim Observations in a Phase I Trial." *Journal of National Cancer Institute* 85 (1993): 611–21.

Haas, C., A. Smith, and A. Lee et al. "Hormone Refractory Prostate Cancer (HRPC): Phase I-II Treatment with Cytoxan, Interferon Alfa 2B and Infusional 5-FU." *Proceedings of American Soc Clinical Oncology* 11 (1992): 214.

Hudes, G., F. Nathan, S. Chapman, R. Greenberg, and C. McAleer. "Combines Antimicrotubule Therapy of Metastatic Prostate Cancer with 96-Hr Paclitaxel and Estramustine: Activity in Hormone-Refractory Disease, *Proceedings of Annual Meeting of American Soc Clinical Oncology* 14, (1995): 237.

Kell W.K., H.I. Scher, and M. Mazumdar et al. "Prostate-Specific Antigen as a Measure of Disease Outcome in Metastatic Hormone-Refractory Prostate Cancer." *Journal Clinical Oncology* 11 (1993): 607–15.

Kennealey, G.T., J.C. Marsh, and D.A. Walsh et al. "Treatment of Advanced Carcinoma of the Prostate with Estramustine and 5-Flourouracil (FU)." *Proceedings American Association Cancer Research and American Soc Clinical Oncology* 19 (1978): 394.

Kobayashi, K., E.E. Vokes, and N.J. Vogelzang et al. "Phase I Study of Suramin Given by Intermittent Infusion Without Adaptive Control in Patients with Advanced Cancer." *Journal of Clinical Oncology* 13 (1995): 2196–07.

Mareel, M.M., G.A. Storme, C.H. Dragonetti, G.K. De Bruyne, B. Hartley-Asp., J.L. Segers, and M.L. Rabaey. "Anti-Invasive Activity of Estramustine on Malignant MO_4 Cells and on DU-145 Human Prostate Carcinoma Cells *In Vitro Cancer Research*" 48, (1986): 1842–49.

O'Bryan, R.M., J.K. Luce, and R.W. Talley et al. "Phase II Evaluation of Adriamycin in Human Neoplasia." *Cancer* 32 (1973): 1–8.

Osborne, C.K., A. Drelichman, and D.D. von Hoff et al. "Mitoxantrone: Modest Activity in a Phase II Trial in Advanced Prostate Cancer." *Cancer Treatment Report* 67 (1983): 1133–35.

Pienta, K.J. and J.E. Lehr. "Inhibition of Prostate Cancer Growth by Estramustine and Etoposide: Evidence for Interaction at the Nuclear Matrix." *Journal of Urology* 149 (1993): 1622–25.

Pienta, K.J., B. Redman, and M. Hussain et al. "Phase II Evaluation of Oral Estramustine and Oral Etoposide in Hormone-Refractory Adenocarcinoma of the Prostate." *Journal Clinical Oncology* 12 (1994): 2005–12.

Reyno, L.M., M.J. Egorin, and M.A. Eisenberger et al. "Development and Validation of a Pharmacokinetically Based Fixed Dosing Scheme for Suramin." *Journal Clinical Oncology* 13 (1995): 2187–95.

Reyno, L.M., M.J. Egorin, and M.A. Eisenberger et al. "Development and Validation of a Pharmacokinetically Based Fixed Dosing Scheme for Suramin." *Proceedings American Soc Clin Oncology* 12 (1993): 135.

Scher, H., A. Yagoda, and R. Watson et al. "Phase II Trial of Doxorubicin in Bidimensionally Measurable Prostatic Adenocarcinoma." *Journal of Urology* 13 (1984): 1099–1102.

Seidman, A.D., H.I. Scher, D. Petrylak, D.D. Dershaw, and T. Curley. "Estramustine and Vinblastine: Use of Prostate Specific Antigen as a Clinical Trial End Point for Hormone Refractory Prostatic Cancer." *Journal of Urology* 147 (1992): 931–34.

Von Roemeling, R., H. Fisher, and R. DeConti et al. "Continuous FUDR for Hormone Refractory Prostate Cancer: A Phase I/II Study." *Proceedings American Soc Clinical Oncology* 10 (1991): 171.

Zhang, Y., P. Talalay, C. G. Cho, and G.H. Posner. "A Major Induces of Anticarcinogenic Protective Enzymes from Broccoli, Isolation and Elucidation of Structure." *Proceedings of National Academy of Sciences*. USA Vol. 89, (March 1992): 2399–2403.

Index

C

Calcitrol, 13
cancer
  green tea as a preventative, 23–24
  green tea as a treatment, 23–24
  lung cancer prevention studies, 13–15
  MCP as a treatment, 19–21
  melanoma cell studies, 19–20
  metastasis, 19
  selenium as a preventative, 16–17
  skin cancer prevention with selenium, 16–17
  types of, 58–59
  vitamin C as a preventative, 12
  vitamin C as a treatment, 12
  See also cancer cells; prostate cancer
cancer cells
  capsule–penetration cells, 93, 97–98
  growth rates, 161
  identifying, 59
  metastasis, 19, 93, 131–132
  PC SPES effect on, 78, 82
  PSA production by, 160
  Rabdosia rebescens effect on, 77
  Scutellaria baicalensis effect on, 76
cancer staging. *See* staging prostate cancer
CAPS questionnaire, 105, 114
capsular penetration, 43, 58, 92–93
  among African American men, 101–102
  biopsies to determine, 58
  radiation treatments affecting, 97–98

carcinomas, effect of *Rabdosia rebescens* on, 77
Caucasian men, prostate cancer characteristics, 101
cells
  lectins, 19
  NK cells, 27
  normal cell destruction by radiation treatments, 165
  red blood cells, 78
  white blood cells, 27, 78, 135
  See also cancer cells
cereal intake and prostate cancer mortality, 30, 31
cervical cancer, effect of *Scutellaria baicalensis* on, 76
chemoprevention, 8–11
  chemopreventive agents, 8–34
  combined with other treatments, 155
  definition, 8
  populations benefitted by, 9–10
  postsurgery, 153
  for watchful waiting, 152
  See also immune enhancers
chemopreventive agents
  characteristics, 10–11
  supplements with chemopreventive properties, 11–34
chemotherapy
  combinations of chemotherapeutic drugs, 139–140, 147–150
  combined with other drugs, 146
  curative chemotherapy, 141
  cytotoxic chemotherapy, 142
  dose intensification, 146